Aspirin Alternatives

The Top Natural Pain-Relieving Analgesics

A Health Learning Handbook

Raymond M. Lombardi, DC, ND, CCN

BL Publications

Temecula, CA

BL Publications, Temecula, CA 92692

Library of Congress Cataloging- In Publication Data

Lombardi, Raymond M., 1960-
   Aspirin alternatives : the top natural pain-relieving analgesics / Raymond M. Lombardi.
   p. cm. -- (A health learning handbook)
   Includes bibliographical references and index.
   ISBN 1-890766-02-X
   1. Analgesics. 2. Pain--Alternative treatment. 3. Herbs--Therapeutic use. 4. Dietary supplements. I. Title. II. Series.
   RM319 .L65 1999
   615'.783--dc21

                                        99-32411
                                          CIP

ISBN: 1-890766-02-X

Printed in the United States of America

First edition, June 1999

Aspirin Alternatives: The Top Natural Pain-Relieving Analgesics is not intended as medical advice. Its intention is solely informational and educational. It is wise to consult your doctor for any illness or medical condition.

Credits:
Typesetting and Cover Design: BL Publications
Editing: Beth Ley Jacobs
Proofreading: Michelle Warnes

Acknowledgment

To my wonderful wife, Peggy.
Thank you for all of your support,
valuable input and keeping the faith.
Onward and upward.

Health Learning Handbooks

These books are designed to provide useful information about ways to improve one's health and well-being. Education about what the body needs to obtain and maintain good health is what we would like to provide.

Good health should not be thought of as absence of disease. We should avoid negative disease oriented thinking and concentrate on what we have to do to remain healthy. Health is maintaining on a daily basis what is essential to the body. Disease is the result of attempting to live without what the body needs. We are responsible for our own health and should take control of it. If we are in control of our health, disease is not likely to take control.

Our health depends on education.

Books in this series include:

Aspirin Alternatives: Top Natural Pain-Relieving Analgesics by Raymond Lombardi, D.C., N.D., C.C.N.

Castor Oil: Its Healing Properties by Beth Ley

CoQ10: All-Around Nutrient For All-Around Health by Beth Ley Jacobs, Ph.D.

Dr. John Willard on Catalyst Altered Water by Beth Ley

Colostrum: Nature's Gift to the Immune System by Beth Ley

DHA: The Magnificent Marine Oil by Beth Ley Jacobs

How to Fight Osteoporosis and Win! The Miracle of Microcrystalline Hydroxyapatite by Beth Ley

PhytoNutrients: Medicinal Nutrients Found in Foods by Beth Ley

MSM: On Our Way Back to Health With Sulfur by Beth Ley

Nature's Road to Recovery: Nutritional Supplements for the Alcoholic and Chemical-dependent by Beth Ley Jacobs, Ph.D.

The Potato Antioxidant: Alpha Lipoic Acid by Beth Ley

The True Vitamin C: Mineral Ascorbates! by Beth Ley Jacobs, Ph.D.

TABLE OF CONTENTS

PREFACE

From the ancients to modern man, pain has been with us throughout our existence. It is one of those aspects of life that we cannot escape. Pain is a universal malady, one that we can expect to experience on numerous occasions during our lifetime and to which no person is immune. In fact, pain could be considered the ultimate aspect of being alive, for "where there is pain, there is life."

Pain is both a blessing and a curse. On the positive side, it is our bodys' way of letting us know when something is wrong and provides us with protection against further damage by pain sensations which cause us to limit motion and activities. Without this critically important mechanism, we would surely perish. But pain, especially unrelieved, chronic pain; can become a serious problem. This type of pain serves neither beneficial purpose nor reason. It is pain that has become unrelenting and debilitating; at times leading to such suffering that a person's life may become shattered and ruined.

Pain, no matter the reason, triggers the immediate desire for relief; preferably the faster the relief, the better. But pain is much more than just a hurtful sensation or a pain syndrome. Pain is a signal, a red flag of alert from our body. More critical than the pain relief is the need to evaluate, understand, treat and correct the underlying cause(s), which have triggered the pain. For both short and long-term relief, the correction of the underlying problem is the most important factor.

Natural approaches to pain relief and pain control have been with us throughout man's recorded history. From the ancient Egyptians to the Chinese culture, natural methods for relieving pain have been documented. It wasn't until the advent of "modern chemical medicine," in this country during the late 1800's and early 1900's that natural approaches were forced out of the mainstream and regaled to the proverbial "back closet." The reasons this occurred are many and beyond the scope of this book. Suffice it to say that the medical and pharmaceutical establishments that came to the forefront during that time period played a significant role in shifting treatment approaches away from "natural medicine." Many natural methods were labeled with such terms as "quackery" and "unscientific," and commonly used natural approaches were derided and dismissed across the spectrum. There can be no doubt that dangerous substances, usually touted as "naturally based," were being hawked by con men and other disreputable persons. The medical establishment made great use of this fact and branded most everything "natural" as useless or dangerous. Ironically, the majority of synthetic, chemical medicines that have been developed have been derived from "natural" plant sources.

In the United States, we are currently undergoing a renaissance in regard to "natural medicine" and the various approaches found under this umbrella term. Usage of Alternative, Natural, Complimentary and Integrative Medicine approaches to health, wellness and disease have been progressing at a fantastic rate. The return to natural methods has been driven by the general public. There is a great deal of dissatisfaction in how medicine is delivered in the United States. For many of you, modern medicine has not provided the needed answers, relief nor resolution of many chronic and debilitating diseases. There is no doubt that medicine in this country focuses on disease and not on wellness and health. Interestingly, modern medicine is facing the same backlash it instigated against natural medicine earlier in this century.

The natural health renaissance has produced an amazing amount of information covering a variety of natural approaches to symptoms and diseases. Research into natural substances and approaches has been going on for a number of years, especially outside of the United States. In the last few years, the amount of research being performed has increased tremendously.

In conjunction with this research, a number of

healthcare professionals from a variety of healthcare disciplines are providing invaluable information in regard to working with natural medicine. Unfortunately, as with so many things in this information age of ours, we are being deluged with too much information; much of it which appears confusing and contradictory. This is further complicated by the fact that many of you are just learning about natural medicine. You don't know which information is right for your particular problem or healthcare needs. You don't have the background nor training to decide which natural approach, either by itself or in combination with others, is needed.

Another critical issue that adds even more complexity to this situation is that many of you are taking over-the-counter and/or prescription medications. It can be extremely dangerous mixing natural substances with synthetic medications. All of these issues makes it very difficult for you to decide what will and won't work for your particular circumstances and what, if any, dangers are involved. How do I know this is occurring? On a daily basis, both inside and outside of my practice, I am bombarded with questions and concerns from the general public concerning natural medicinal approaches. It was from this that I realized a reference type of book was needed to help you sort through the minefield of natural health.

In my practice, I deal with the issue of pain and pain relief everyday. I have learned from my patients the harsh realities of living with pain, both acute and chronic, and the struggles involved to relieve it and resolve the conditions which cause it. It was from these experiences that I decided to focus this book on natural pain relieving methods.

It is my hope that you find this book an excellent resource for background information and as a quick reference when you need to treat pain and pain-related conditions.

To Your Good Health and Happiness. Naturally.

Dr. Raymond M. Lombardi

HOW TO USE THIS BOOK

As I was writing this book, one factor remained at the forefront of my mind. I realize that when a person is experiencing pain, the first consideration is to decrease and relieve the pain in the fastest manner possible. However, depending on the location and cause of the pain and many other elements, your pain relief will vary from immediate to more slowly resolving. In this regard, it makes no difference whether you are using natural approaches, over-the-counter or prescription medications. Remember, while the sensation of "pain" is of immediate concern, the important point is to resolve the underlying condition. Beware! This is a theme that will be repeated throughout this book! It is that important! Overall, this book has been designed as both a background reference text and for quick access to specific complaints and conditions.

This book is setup in a simple, three-section format. Sections I and II cover important background information and are described in more detail below. Please take time to review both sections. Perhaps the most important section for your use is Section III. This is the area in which you will turn too for information in regard to natural, pain relieving substances and methods. And at the end of Section III there is a quick access chart for pain relief that has been provided for immediate information on a variety of conditions.

Section I discusses basic background information in regard to pain mechanisms and its pathways, the body's production of pain relievers and the dangers of both prescription and over-the-counter pain medications. This section will give you a basic understanding of our body's response to pain including the different types and aspects of pain and our body's natural pain suppression mechanisms. It will discuss some of the dangers related to traditional pain relievers and the reasons we take them. Finally, other reasons that pain relievers are taken will be discussed.

Section II provides you with information on our return to natural approaches and the standard and non-standard approaches to natural pain relief. This section provides the rational for utilizing natural approaches to both pain relief and in resolving the conditions which are creating the pain sensation. Descriptions are provided concerning the importance and various ways in which natural procedures can be used.

The most important section for your reference and usage is **Section III**. This area of the book will provide descriptions and background information of the natural substances and methods that can be used for pain relief. At the end of this section is a quick reference chart for pain remedies, complaints and underlying conditions. Section III is composed of **Three Essential Modules** designed to help you quickly get the answers you need.

Module One, entitled **"Natural Substances,"** provide a general listing of the various substances which can be used for pain relief. Module One includes substances which can be taken orally and/or are used topically. This module contains different categories which includes: Vitamins, Minerals, Other Supplements, Enzymes, Amino Acids, Topicals, Herbals, and Homeopathic substances.

Module Two is entitled **"Natural Physical Methods."** This module lists, describes and discusses the various physical approaches to pain relief, such as chiropractic, acupuncture and others. You will utilize these two modules as a point of entry to provide you with in-depth information on the natural substances and methods.

Module Three, which is at the end of Section Three, is entitled **"Pain Resolving Strategies."** It is a quick access/reference chart which has been set up to provide you with listings of a variety of pain complaints, conditions and the natural substances and methods that can be used to resolve them. This chart has been designed in a column method with three specific categories. The following is the format:

Category/Column One is called **"Pain Complaints and Disorders."** *It lists a number of pain complaints, problems and conditions which have pain as part of their presentation.*

Category/Column Two has been designed to provide you with immediate pain relief solutions whenever possible for the problems listed in column one. This category has been entitled **"Immediate Pain Relief."**

Category/Column Three is entitled "**Secondary Pain Relieving Methods"** *for complaints in which natural approaches do not lend themselves to immediate pain control, you will be referred to Category/Column Three. This category will provide the best solutions for stimulating the quickest resolution of the underlying conditions. This third category is critical for long term relief.*

For Categories Two and Three in Module Three, I have provided as many solutions for you as possible keeping space and materials in consideration.

In Modules One and Two, when necessary, precautions may be listed. **Please review information under this heading prior to using natural approaches.** *This is of critical importance! There may be side effects, contraindications, drug interactions, etc., which need to be addressed. In Module Three, there are conditions, diseases and circumstances which may require* <u>immediate medical attention.</u> *If this is indicated in the book, please act accordingly. In general, conditions which are medical emergencies have not been included in this book because of the need for immediate medical intervention. However, a particular pain complaint may be the early sign of a serious disease. It is always a good idea to be evaluated by a healthcare professional for conditions which are not of an obvious nature or cause. Becoming well-informed in all aspects of health care, both medical and natural-based, is essential to becoming an educated health care consumer.*

At the end of the book, you will find a **Recommended Reading List** *to give you further information on various natural substances and natural meth-*

ods. Why is this reference list important? This book has been designed as a "Quick Access Manual," with specific listings of substances and methods which can provide both immediate and long-term pain relief. It was not designed as an all-encompassing reference text, especially in regard to the huge amount of material currently available regarding natural medicine.

Finally, in all cases the beginning of good health starts with the basics: Correct whole food eating and eating patterns, general supplementation, proper water intake, rest, and exercise. All of these are of critical importance. However, due to the limitation of space, unless indicated as a treatment approach, I will not be focusing on these aspects. Take time to study and learn about each of these. Without the fundamentals, you will have difficulty in maintaining good health and resolving any health problems.

The Causes and Affects Of Pain

What is pain? Dorland's Medical Dictionary states that pain is "a feeling of distress, suffering, or agony, caused by stimulation of specialized nerve endings." A very clinical way of stating that our bodies have an incredible system available to us, using a "pain sensation" to signal us when damage is occurring. This is an important concept because many diseases and afflictions of the body cause pain.

The primary purpose of pain is its function as a protective mechanism for the body. It is part of the body's warning system. Pain usually is an indication that tissues have been irritated or damaged. For example, you may have burned yourself or sprained your ankle. However, there are times that pain can arise when there is no apparent damage or injury to the body.

Pain is an amazingly complex subject. First off, pain is an unpleasant "sensation" that we experience. The "pain experience" occurs in a number of ways and has many aspects to it. These include such things as a person's anticipation of pain, pain expectation, previous pain experience, emotional and psychological factors, cultural differences, the individual's tolerances and capacity to deal with the pain, etc. Pain is very subjective and individually based. What one person may experience as moderate or even excruciating pain, another person may experience as a mild pain and discomfort. This is an extreme example, but I have been amazed at the individual differences and tolerances I have witnessed in patients in my practice. It is important to understand that pain is not always what appears on the surface.

To provide you with a basic understanding of pain, we must begin with a brief discussion of the pain pathways in our body. While this material may seem difficult to understand without a medical background, a basic understanding of how our body stimulates, derives and interprets pain is very important.

The pain pathways discussed below are only one physical aspect of the complex experience that we call pain. I have made every effort to take this established clinical knowledge and put it into understandable terms; however, some words and statements don't lend themselves to simple terms.

To understand the pain pathways, we must have a basic understanding of the nervous system and how it functions. According to Dorland's Medical Dictionary, the nervous system is "the organ system which, along with the endocrine system, correlates the adjustments and reactions of the organism to its internal and external environment, comprising the central and peripheral nervous systems." In simple terms, the nervous system provides most of the control functions for the body; including both sensory and motor functions, as it responds and reacts to the environment outside and inside of us. For the purposes of this book, we will focus on those portions of the nervous system

16

that relate to the experience of pain.

To best describe how our bodies come to respond to a "pain" stimulus, we begin with the pain receptors. Pain receptors are specialized sensory nerve endings that responds to various stimuli (such as a burning candle) by responding with a pain signal. Think of a piece of thread (the free nerve ending/receptor) that is lying in the skin or within a muscle. These "receptors" are spread throughout our skin, organs, bone coverings, arterial walls, joint surfaces, muscles and ligaments, etc.

When something occurs, such as trauma or damage, a signal is relayed to these specialized receptors that is interpreted as a "pain stimulus." At this point, the pain stimulus is transmitted along specialized sensory nerves to the spinal cord and up to the brain, where the pain stimulus is processed and a response is provided back to the various structures which need to initiate an action (such as moving our hand away from the flame).

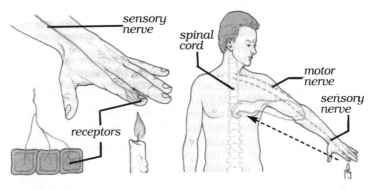

Receptors in the fingertips detect heat/pain. Signals are sent along a sensory nerve to the spinal cord. The signals arriving in the spinal cord pass instantaneously to a motor nerve that connects a muscle in the arm. The signals received cause the muscles to contract moving the arm away from the source of pain.

The following is an example of the pain response process. The following scenario will provide you with an understanding of this process: You are walking barefooted and step on a nail. The "negative stimulus" is the nail penetrating the skin of your foot.

1. The "pain receptors" in the skin of your foot are activated by the penetrating nail. This stimulation is translated into a "pain signal" which travels through the afferent (sensory) pathway to the spinal cord.

2. Within the spinal cord, the pain signal is sent through more sensory tracts to the brain, which becomes aware and analyzes the pain stimulus.

3. The brain then sends an outgoing signal to various areas of the body which initiates a response. The head, neck, arms, trunk and opposite leg (causing muscular reactive movements), and the tongue, throat and respiration (gasp of pain or an exclamation), all may respond.

4. Further, a signal is sent back down the spinal cord and out the "efferent" (motor) pathway to the "effectors" (motor receptors in the muscles); in this case, to the muscles of the leg and foot which stepped on the nail.

5. The final reaction is the sharp withdrawal of the foot from the nail (the pain stimulus).

The response time in this entire scenario is instantaneous. It is interpreted by the body and reacted to so fast that we are already pulling our foot away from the nail before we actually have conscious recognition of what actually has occurred.

Pain receptors are located all over our body. Most of our deep tissues are not heavily supplied with these or other types of pain receptors; however, there are enough to create a pain stimulus. There are essentially three types of pain receptors: Mechanosensitive receptors, stimulated by mechanical stress or damage; Thermosensitive receptors, stimulated by heat or cold; and Chemosensitive receptors, stimulated by various chemical substances which are irritating. An example of each of these is as follows:

1. Mechanosensitive receptors: You suffer an ankle sprain while playing soccer. The mechanical stress and damage to the muscles, ligaments and ankle joint stimulates this type of receptor and you experience pain.

2. Thermosensitive receptors: You take a pan of boiling soup off the stove and accidentally brush your hand against the pan's surface; or after a night of freezing weather, you brush your hand up against a frozen pipe. In both cases, the sensitivity of these receptors to heat and cold will activate the pain response. You will experience pain and immediately withdraw your hand.

3. Chemosensitive receptors: You are cleaning your car battery and some of the acid gets on you hand. The acid will stimulate this type of receptor and you will experience pain.

As discussed previously, once the pain receptors have received a stimulus, they send a pain signal along the afferent (sensory) nerve pathway of pain fibers back to the spinal cord. There is an important aspect to this pain signal and the response of the pain fibers. The pain fibers contain two components: "Fast" pain fibers and "Slow" pain fibers. This is important because we end up with a double system of pain innervation; one which gives us a fast "pricking type" of pain and the other a slower, "burning" sensation of pain. The "pricking" pain tells us very quickly that damage may be occurring and thus we react to stop it. The "burning" pain tends to become more and more painful over time, is most apparent after tissue damage and tends to linger.

At the spinal cord, the pain stimulus enters the cord and travels along specified "sensory spinal tracts" to the brain. These spinal cord tracts are specific to the transfer of the pain signal and are very complex. An important consideration of these tracts is that the "intensity" of the pain sensation can be modified as it travels to the brain; either as a decreased or increased pain signal. The pain signal is eventually transmitted to the brain where it is received, interpreted and an appropriate response sent back to the body to initiate a specific action.

Please realize that the above explanation is a simplistic rendition of this incredibly complex system. The pain sensation and response is very involved and tends to integrate directly and indirectly, many other aspects of the nervous system. Our bodies have a magnificent network to provide us with pain sensations and a way to respond to them.

The pain sensation is as varied as it is complex. Pain can occur in one area, multiple areas, and radiate from one site to another. Pain is most often classified based on its duration and whether its source is somatic or visceral. Pain duration is described as:

- **Acute** (new, immediate or recent)

- **Prolonged or subacute** (lasting days to weeks)

- **Chronic** (ongoing, lasting months to years)

Acute pain is usually of a short time frame, tends to be protective in nature and is usually not associated with significant tissue damage. Prolonged pain is the most common form and is always associated with tissue injury and inflammation. Chronic pain typically is just the opposite of acute. It can be of unlimited duration, is usually not protective to the body, and can be associated with significant tissue damage. In some chronic pain cases, the damage may have been resolved but the pain syndrome continues. Chronic pain is defined as pain lasting longer than six months.

Pain can strike different body tissues and regions. Terms have been defined to identify particular structures. The term "somatic" relates to the skin, muscles, ligaments, joints, connective tissue, etc. It is characterized as being localized, meaning you can pinpoint the area from which the pain is coming from. An example of this type of pain would be from spraining the right ankle. When you sprain your right ankle, you know that you have hurt and damaged the right ankle.

Visceral pain, on the other hand, is diffuse (spread out) and difficult to localize. It can be from organs or deep lying, non-organ structures and can refer pain to the skin. An example would be pain from the gall bladder. That pain is spread across the right mid to low abdomen, and can refer pain to the low and mid back and down into the groin on the right side.

Pain can be described in many ways: Aching, throbbing, burning, deep, stabbing, dull, sharp, etc. Pain descriptions, to limit confusion, have been placed into three specific categories. They are:

● **Pricking Pain** is experienced when we stick ourselves with a sharp object or cut our skin.

● **Burning Pain** occurs when we burn our skin.

● **Aching Pain** is a deep type of pain that can vary from an annoyance to severe pain.

Pain descriptions are very important in identifying the pain syndrome. Different types of pain are experienced with different conditions. Establishing and learning your particular pain pattern is important in developing a treatment program specific to your needs.

So you now have an idea of how pain works and how it is categorized. But how do we feel and experience pain? As headaches, neck and back pain, joint pain, abdominal pain, menstrual pain, reproductive pain, pain from trauma and injury, organ pain (such as from the gallbladder or liver), disease pain (such as from cancer or arthritis), etc. Pain is such a common malady that we have labeled areas of the affected part of the body with a pain title that is descriptive to that part or area: Headaches, low back pain, etc. Pain is not particular, it can strike all parts of our bodies. What is important, is to learn and understand the causes of pain. With this knowledge, you and your health care professional can evaluate and treat not only the pain itself, but the underlying cause that has triggered the pain response.

Our Natural Production Of Pain Relievers

When pain occurs, the desire and need for pain relief becomes all important. We may not even realize that the body suffers many aches and pains each day in which we may experience as simple soreness, or have no pain experience at all. Our bodies, being the miracle machines they are, have a built-in mechanism to deal with pain. This capability is critical to our very survival. Without this ability, we would surely perish. While we do not currently understand and know of all the possible substances which make up this pain relief system, science has discovered a few substances within this group. These substances are called endorphins, enkephalins and substance P. The following is an explanation and description of these substances. Don't let the medical information in this portion stop you from reading through the material. It is background information, so work through it as best as possible.

These substances are termed neurotransmitters, and are found in specific areas of the brain and possibly in other areas of the body. A neurotransmitter (NT) is defined as a chemical that is selectively released from a nerve terminal by an action potential, then interacts with a specific receptor on an adjacent structure and produces a specific physiologic response. The endorphins have been found in abundance in the hypothalamus and in the pituitary gland. The enkephalins are found mainly in those areas of the brain associated with pain control, including the periventricular area, the periaqueductal gray , the midline raphe nuclei, the substantia gelatinosa of the dorsal horns in the spinal cord, and the intralaminar nuclei of the thalamus.

Endorphins are believed to bind to opiate receptors in various areas of the brain and thereby raise the pain threshold. Though several different types of endorphins have been isolated, the most potent and presumably most important is B-endorphin.

Enkephalins are believed to have potent, opiate-like effects; thus leading to analgesia. Enkephalins have been defined into two naturally occurring types called methionine enkephalin and leucine enkephalin. Substance P is a peptide and is the transmitter of many central neurons (e.g. dorsal root ganglia, basal ganglia, hypothalamus). Its synthesis and fate are similar to those of the endorphins and enkephalins. All of these substances have been found at different points in the analgesic system.

Perhaps the best way of understanding how this internal pain relief system works is to look at how our bodies respond after moderate muscular exercise. This can be from weight training, aerobic exercise or just plain old-fashioned labor, like digging. All of these exercises cause us to utilize our muscular system and activate a series of biochemical reactions. The usage of our muscles, especially with moderate or sustained activity, triggers the release of the natural, opiate-like chemicals within our bodies. Why is this important? Because without these substances, we would be in agony from the muscle usage!

It has been proposed that these substances may also reduce both anxiety and depression by their actions. They may do a great many things, but to date, only limited amounts of information have been gathered concerning these incredible chemicals. Watch for future information concerning these substances. As science continues to unravel their mysteries, we may find them playing an important role in future pain management.

The Dangers Of Prescription and Over-The-Counter Medications

If you are like most in this society, when pain rears its ugly head, you immediately turn to some form of pain reliever. The kind of pain reliever that we take can depend on a variety of factors. These include the types of and causes of the pain, whether it is from acute injury or chronic disease processes, inflammation, swelling, fever, etc.

Pain relievers (also known as "analgesics"), can be broken down into two basic categories: Over-the-counter pain relievers and prescription pain relievers. Within these two categories are sub-groups which we will discuss. The over-the-counter variety are those that are easily accessible and do not require a prescription from a doctor to obtain. They are available from pharmacies, grocery and convenience stores, etc. Included in this group are aspirin, ibuprofen (Motrin, Advil), acetaminophen (Tylenol), ketoprofen (Orudis), and naproxen (Aleve). These drugs are typically used as analgesics and/or for there anti-inflammatory capability (inflammation reducers). These types of analgesics have mild to moderate pain relieving properties.

The second type of analgesics are only available by prescription from a physician. Included in this group are such drugs as Vicodin, Neurontin, Codeine, and Darvocet. These tend to be more potent in their pain relieving properties, may have addictive qualities, and are typically prescribed for moderate to severe pain.

There are many synthetic pain relievers available

to the public and we are taking them in amounts measured in tons each year. Just how popular are these over-the-counter and prescription analgesics? You may be shocked to learn that we spend billions of dollars on them each year!

When the discussion of pain relief comes up with my patients, I will be the first to admit that I am an advocate for both pain relief and pain control. I do not believe that suffering, whether of a short duration or prolonged, is beneficial to the healing process nor to the person. Typically, regardless of whether it is traditional western medicine or from an alternative care standpoint, the first point of treatment is to begin procedures which will provide pain relief. At times, this may indeed involve the use of "synthetic" analgesics.

These analgesics can and do provide some level of pain relief in many cases. So if they work, why not take them? The problem with this approach is that it does not consider the negative side effects of these medicines nor their general abuse and misuse. Our society has taken to using these pain medications for "every ache and pain" and unfortunately, for a variety of other ills in which these medicines may or may not have any therapeutic value.

Remember, pain relievers seek to "handle" pain, **not correct the underlying problem**. Take a moment and think about this statement! It is critical to understand that pain relievers are a superficial "band-aid;" one that is designed to provide prophylactic relief, not resolve the cause of the pain itself. While part of the overall treatment program needs to integrate pain management, merely controlling and relieving the pain will not correct the cause of the pain. In the United States, we have become so used to "taking the pain away," we forget that the pain would not be there if not

> # Pain relievers do not correct the
> # underlying problem!

for some type of underlying problem!

An important aspect of modern medicine is the concept of "benefit versus risk" in the application of drug therapy. In simple terms, this treatment approach weighs the possible benefit that a medication may infer to a patient for the treatment of a particular disease or condition against the potential and real, negative side effects that can result from the usage of the medication.

Critical to drug therapy is the understanding of the chemistry, biochemistry, pharmacology, and toxicology of the different medications and their interactions with the human body. The pain medications we are discussing are synthetically derived and produced through chemical manipulation in laboratories. Why is this important? Inherent in this chemical process is that synthetically produced drugs, by their very nature, are intended to create a reaction within the body; in this case, pain relief. It is important to remember that pain medications are designed to impact a single or a few specific chemical receptors that induce a greater response in the brain and nervous system.

Unfortunately, these chemicals have both direct and indirect effects on cells and other areas unrelated to their intended points of interaction. It is from the direct reaction to these chemicals and their interaction within the closed biochemical environment of our bodies, that side effects develop. This is part of the negative aspects of modern drug therapy in which there can be a spectrum of consequences ranging from mild side effects to the extreme; at times leading even to death.

This should be of grave concern to us all. All of the available pain-relieving drugs have side effects associated with them, side effects that have been well established through medical research and study. The terrifying reality is that most of the general public remains largely uneducated concerning these side effects. Even worse, are those people who are unconcerned about the side effects of pain medications. How have we come to this place?

Each medication comes with an information sheet, either within the package or from the pharmacist. This insert sheet provides facts concerning the medication, including the chemistry, usage, dosages, side effects, contraindications, cautions, warnings, etc. I have found that the information sheets provided by the pharmacist tend to be easier to understand and are written in more understandable terms. Regardless, many do not bother to read the information that is provided with these medications. I suspect that even for those that do read the material, many don't understand its importance nor the risk factors involved. If we are not informed or educated concerning the medicines we take, how can we possibly understand their dangers?

Then there is the misuse, and in some cases, abuse of the medications we take. How many of you take your medications, whether over-the-counter or prescription, as prescribed or directed? The fact is, many people do not take their medications as directed. Why does this occur? There are a number of reasons for this phenomenon. In regard to pain medication, the usual reason is that the given dose is not proving effec-

> **Do you read AND understand the chemistry, usage, dosages, side effects, contraindications, cautions, warnings, etc., of ALL the medications you take or are prescribed?**

tive or working fast enough. Our desire for immediate, complete pain relief can lead us to take more of a medication than is directed. This unfortunately fits with the "more is better" concept which pervades our society. This attitude certainly applies to our over-usage of medications.

Part of this same problem is taking medications more frequently than directed. This is especially true of pain relievers. Some medications have very specific time frames for usage and with good reason. An example would be taking the directed dose of over-the-counter Advil every four to six hours. But due to pain levels, we decide to take the same dose, but at an increased frequency of every two hours. This can be extremely dangerous as toxic levels can build up within the body.

Another potentially dangerous area is mixing different pain medications with other pain medications or with other medications, either at the same time or switching back and forth between various types. Because of potential chemical interactions and toxicity levels that can build up in the bloodstream, mixing pain medications, and any other medications, can be extremely dangerous unless directed by your doctor. I suggest that consumers verify all medication information with a pharmacist so that no mistakes happen when more than one medication is being used. There should also be concerns in regard to the elderly, the pregnant, food interactions, drug allergies and hyper-sensitivity reactions, etc. The reality is there are many inherent dangers in taking pain medications, and these dangers are real and well established.

An area that most of us accept without too much thought or consideration is the impact that advertising has had on each of us. We live in the information age. The various media forms, including print, television, radio and the internet, all provide us with vast amounts of information everyday. In fact, on average, Americans are exposed to 270 advertisements each day! This arena is well utilized for advertising pain medications. Not a day goes by that we do not encounter some type of advertising extolling the virtues of pain-relievers. In a typical evening of television view-ing, we may see as many as six or more ads for these products. This daily bombardment tells us to "get rid of the pain, you don't have to suffer," etc. This has had serious negative effects on our society.

We have become numb and accepting to the potential serious side effects of these medications in part because they are so grossly over-promoted. Our perceptions and beliefs that these medications are "safe" are based more on aggressive advertising than on the established facts.

Even worse, new advertising laws have allowed the pharmaceutical companies even more aggressive approaches to advertising; using celebrity stars to pro-mote their wares. Along with this, they are also required to list some of the side effects. Interestingly, the terminology used are statements like: "a low inci-dence of side effects have occurred including..." The perception is that these medication's side effects are

> ## *Aggressive advertising has mislead us to believing pain relievers are harmless!*

"normal and safe." When did it become normal to have any side effects? How can any negative reaction in our bodies be considered safe? Regardless of possible short term benefits, any negative side effects must be seriously considered prior to usage. This is especially true of pain medications which are so overused in this country.

So, how aggressively do we attack our various "aches and pains?" In the United States, we consume over 19 billion aspirin tablets each year – over 15 tons each day! Yearly sales for Ibuprofen and Acetaminophen are well over $2 billion. However, there is a price to pay for our pain relief and it comes in the form of damage to our bodies.

Are these "side effects" of real concern? Absolutely! There are both potential and well-established, dangerous reactions to pain medications. These side effects may be mild or severe. Liver damage, blood cell destruction, drowsiness, insomnia, neuropathy, dependence and addictions are just a few of the side effects of pain medications.

The following are some of the known side effects of a few of the common over-the-counter and prescription pain relievers.

Included in this group of pain relievers are non-steroidal anti-inflammatories (NSAIDS). NSAIDS are a general term used for a group of drugs that are effective in reducing inflammation and pain. These include aspirin, ibuprofen, ketoprofen and naproxen sodium.

NSAIDS are generally quickly absorbed into the bloodstream. Pain and fever relief can occur within one hour of taking the first dose and can last four to six hours. This group makes up the majority of over-the-counter pain medications.

Side Effects of Common Over-The-Counter Medications:

From: The Pill Book Guide To Over-The-Counter Medications; Editor-in-chief Robert P. Rapp, Pharm. D.

These side effects are "possible;" meaning they can and do occur, but not with every person. Side effects are more likely with over-usage and abuse of these medications. You will note some basic commonalties between the different medications listed.

Acetaminophen: (Tylenol)
Most common: Lightheadedness.
Less common: Trembling and pain in lower back or side.
Rare: Extreme fatigue, rash, itching, or hives, sore throat or fever, unexplained bleeding or bruising, anemia, yellowing of the skin or eyes, blood in urine, painful or frequent urination and decreased output of urine volume. In doses of more than 4 grams per day (4000 mg), acetaminophen is potentially toxic to the liver. Use acetaminophen with caution if you have kidney or liver disease or viral infections of the liver.

Aleve (Naproxen sodium):
Most common: Gastrointestinal (GI) problems (e.g. constipation, indigestion, heartburn, nausea, diarrhea, and stomach irritation).

Less common: Stomach ulcers, GI bleeding, loss of appetite, hepatitis, gallbladder problems, painful urination, poor kidney function, kidney inflammation, blood in the urine, dizziness, fainting, and nervousness.

Rare: Severe allergic reactions, including closing of the throat, fever and chills, changes in liver function, jaundice, kidney failure, ringing in the ears, and blurred vision.

Aspirin (Acetylsalicylic acid):

Common: Nausea, upset stomach, heartburn, loss of appetite, and appearance of small amounts of blood in the stool.

Rare: Hives, rashes, liver damage, fever, thirst and difficulties with vision.

Aspirin may contribute to the formation of stomach ulcers and bleeding. People who are allergic to aspirin and those with a history of nasal polyps, asthma, or rhinitis may experience breathing difficulty and a stuffy nose.

Another precautions with Aspirin is that it should not be taken by children under 16 years of age unless it is recommended by a doctor. This is because of the risk of a rare complication called Reyes Syndrome. This disease, occurring mostly in children, causes damage to the nerves, brain and liver. In about 30% of the cases, it is fatal. Aspirin is associated with gastrointestinal (GI) irritation, erosion, and bleeding and should not be used by individuals with a GI bleeding disorder or a history of peptic ulcers. Aspirin has been shown to be harmful to the developing fetus, and should not be taken by pregnant women. Aspirin should not be taken by patients who are taking anticoagulation (blood thinning) drugs. Aspirin use should be stopped immediately if there is continuous stomach pain, dizziness, hearing loss and ringing or buzzing in the ears.

Ibuprofen: (Motrin, Advil)

Most common: GI problems (e.g. indigestion, heartburn, nausea, diarrhea, stomach irritation).

Less common: Stomach ulcers, GI bleeding, loss of appetite, hepatitis, gallbladder attacks, painful urination, poor kidney function, kidney inflammation, blood in the urine, dizziness, fainting, and nervousness.

Rare: Severe allergic reactions, including closing of the throat, fever, and chills, changes in liver function, jaundice, and kidney failure; ringing in the ears, blurred vision.

Ketoprofen: (Orudis KT)

Most common: Stomach upset or irritation, diarrhea, nausea, vomiting, constipation, stomach gas, and loss of appetite.

Less common: Stomach ulcers, GI bleeding, hepatitis, gallbladder attacks, painful urination, poor kidney function, kidney inflammation, blood and protein in the urine, dizziness, fainting, nervousness, depression, hallucinations, confusion, disorientation, lightheadedness, tingling in the hands or feet, itching, increased sweating, dry nose and mouth, heart palpitations, chest pain, difficulty breathing, and muscle cramps.

Rare: Severe allergic reactions, including closing of the throat, fever and chills, headache, visual disturbances, swelling in the hands or feet, changes in liver function, jaundice, and kidney failure.

Side Effects of Common Prescription Pain Medications:

From: The Essential Guide To Prescription Drugs by James J. Rybacki, Pharm. D. and James W. Long, M.D.

These medications are classed as narcotics and opioids and are only available by prescription. The side effects with this group are presented in a different way because of the strength and action of these medications. These medications may be taken or prescribed by themselves or combined with other analgesics and medications.

Codeine:

Possible side effects (natural, expected, and unavoidable drug actions): Drowsiness, lightheadedness, dry mouth, urinary retention, constipation (frequent and dose related).

Mild adverse effects: Allergic reactions, skin rash, hives, itching, dizziness, impaired concentration, sensation of drunkenness, confusion, depression, blurred or double vision, nausea and vomiting.

Serious adverse effects: Allergic reactions, anaphylaxis, severe skin reactions, idiosyncratic reactions, delirium, hallucinations, excitement, increased sensitivity to pain after the analgesic effect has born off, seizures (rare), impaired breathing (dose related), liver toxicity and porphyria.

Opiates have a variety of effects on sexual response. These may range from blunting of sexual response to increased response if anxiety has been a factor inhibiting response.

Other adverse effects: Paradoxical behavioral disturbances (which may suggest a psychotic disorder), reduced blood platelet count, increased blood amylase and lipase levels.

Hydrocodone (Vicodin):

Possible side effects (natural, expected, and unavoidable drug actions): Drowsiness, lightheadedness, dry mouth, urinary retention, constipation. Possible adverse effects (unusual, unexpected, and infrequent reactions)

Mild adverse effects: Allergic reactions: skin rash, hives, itching; dizziness, impaired concentration, sensation of drunkenness, confusion, depression, blurred or double vision, facial flushing, sweating; nausea, vomiting and abnormal constriction of the pupils of the eye.

Serious adverse effects: Allergic reactions, anaphylaxis, severe skin reactions, idiosyncratic reactions, delirium, hallucinations, excitement, increased sensitivity to pain after the analgesic effect has worn off, seizures, impaired breathing (respiratory depression), liver or kidney toxicity, psychological and physical dependence, blunting of sexual response or drive, increased blood amylase and lipase levels.

Oxycodone (Percocet/Percodan):

Possible side effects (natural, expected and unavoidable drug actions): Drowsiness, lightheadedness, dry mouth, urinary retention, constipation.

Mild adverse effects: Allergic reactions, skin rash, hives, itching; idiosyncratic reactions, skin rash and itching when combined with dairy products, dizziness, sensation of drunkenness, depression, blurred or double vision, nausea and vomiting.

Serious adverse effects: Impaired breathing, abnormal body movements, blunted sexual responses.

Possible effect of long term use: Psychological and physical dependence, chronic constipation.

Use of Pain Relievers Creates Numerous Health Problems

After reading this list of potential, possible and real side effects from over-the-counter and prescription medications, it should be obvious that these medications pose the serious potential to harm us. What this list does not include is the general effects on the different systems of the body that is producing these "side effects."

For example, chronic constipation may result from pain medication use. If our elimination system is compromised and becomes sluggish, what are the effects "upstream" from the colon? Does the constipation change the fluid balance in both the colon and small intestines? The pH balance? The flora balance in the small intestine? The digestive and proteolytic enzymes which are critical to digestion? I believe that any impact in one part of a system will have either a direct and/or indirect impact on the rest of the system.

Further, in looking at the anatomy and physiology of the body, it is apparent that loss of optimum function in part or all of a system will in turn effect other systems and the human body as a whole. So, is it worth it? It all comes down to risk versus benefit. Consider these listed side effects. These medications should only be used as a last resort, when natural approaches have proven to be ineffective to either control the pain or resolve the underlying condition that is causing the pain.

There will certainly be times in which these pain medications are necessary; serious conditions like cancer, in which the pain can become severe and unrelenting. The point here is that it is always better to utilize natural methods which have minimal to no side effects as the first line of attack. Lets save these potent medications for the times we truly need them.

Why We Take Pain Medication

In our society today, we take pain relievers for a number of reasons. Pain relief is usually the primary one, but analgesics are also used for a variety of other conditions and purposes; some reasonable and others that are not. Pain relievers, thanks to their chemical makeup and pharmacological actions, can provide responses within the body beyond that of pain relief. They are used to reduce fevers, to thin the blood, as preventative care for the heart, etc. However, pain relievers are used in cases which have minimal value in regard to their pain relieving properties.

One of the first examples that comes to mind is the use of pain relievers in nighttime sleep medications. Typically, these over-the-counter medicines combine some type of analgesic with an anti-histamine; all with the intent of helping us get to and stay asleep. On the surface, this appears to be a good combination. But is it? What benefit do we garner from introducing a pain reliever into the body as an aid to sleep? If we are in pain and that pain is impacting our sleep pattern, then the usage of a pain reliever might be warranted. Yet, there are natural pain relievers which would be just as effective without the side effects that can come from the over-the-counter medications.

More importantly, when people usually take these particular combinations, there is no pain involved at all. (I also have concerns in regard to the chronic usage of anti-histamines as sleep aids, but that is beyond the scope of this book.) If there is no pain syndrome and the analgesic medication is not specifically oriented for a needed physiologic reason, why put our body into the position of having to deal with it?

To understand the reasons this occurs, one need only look at our society's usage and perspective concerning medications. Sadly, our society has become indoctrinated in the "need" of medications, even when their value is minimal or does not exist. I know that the pharmaceutical conglomerates would vigorously deny this statement, but their perspective is driven as much, if not more, by economics, rather than just the publics healthcare needs.

I have listed below some of the pain relieving medications that are used for other purposes. This is not an all-encompassing list, but placed here to give you a little perspective. The main alternate usages for pain medications are usually for their anti-inflammatory effects (inflammation reducing) and anti-pyretic effects (relieving or reducing fevers). Another usage, especially with aspirin, is as a blood thinner. Because of this capability, it is used as a preventive measure for certain cardiovascular diseases.

Aleve: (Naproxen sodium) Anti-inflammatory, menstrual cramps, and fever reducer.

Arthropan: (Choline salicylate) Analgesic and fever reducer.

Aspirin: Anti-inflammatory and anti-coagulant.

Doan's: (Magnesium salicylate) Fever reducer.

Excedrin Aspirin-Free Analgesic Caplets: (Acetaminophen and caffeine) Fever reducer, mild diuretic and central nervous system (CNS) stimulant.

Excedrin Extra Strength: (Aspirin, acetaminophen and caffeine) Anti-inflammatory, anti-coagulant, central nervous system stimulant and diuretic.

Ibuprofen: Anti-inflammatory, reducer of fever and menstrual cramps.

As you can see from this group, pain relievers do have other capabilities. However, there are many natural substances that can perform many of the same functions; especially in regard to anti-inflammatory and muscular cramping effects. These could be utilized to provide the same results without the negative side effects. For more information, please consult Section Three and the Reading List at the end of this book.

The Change Back To Natural Remedies

Our society is at an interesting crossroads in regard to medicine. Many Americans are choosing to use "natural-based" approaches to their healthcare. Even the mainstay of the medical community, the *New England Journal of Medicine*, has been forced to deal with this phenomenon. They did so by publishing an issue in 1998 which dealt exclusively with alternative medicine. The fact that there interpretations and conclusions in that issue left much to be desired is not the point; what is important, is that recognition of what is occurring in the United States has reached mainstream medicine. Make no mistake, the medical establishment has sat up and taken notice. That being said, don't expect the medical community to suddenly become ardent supporters of this new dynamic in healthcare. While alternative medicine is getting a lot of media press, there continues to be as much resistance, and in certain quarters, even more resistance than ever before. There are loud demands from the medical community that "alternative medicine" provide both research and clinical studies as to their effectiveness, and to place themselves under rigorous scientific scrutiny and critiques. This is the same scrutiny that pharmaceutical medicines and medical procedures are subjected to. The stated reason is that "alternative medicine" needs to prove its effectiveness, capabilities, usages, contraindications, toxicity levels, side effects, safety, etc.

While I am very supportive of the need for clinical research, clinical studies and scientific reviews of alternative medicine, I have major reservations as to the validity and findings that may come from such an undertaking. The results will depend on who is doing the research and the clinical studies. There has been extensive research and clinical studies performed on many natural substances and alternative medicine approaches outside of the United States. Research of alternative medicine in this country has been limited because the medical establishment in this country has, for decades, put roadblocks in the way of legitimate research and clinical studies. Would I trust the medical community's findings concerning alternative medicine. The answer is a resounding NO! But let's take this a step further and move away from an antagonistic point of view.

According to their own research, approximately 60 to 75 percent of mainstream medical approaches, especially in regard to medicines, are not clinically validated for their effectiveness and usage. Who does the majority of the testing and clinical research on medicines? The pharmaceutical companies which produce them. The very people who have an immense economic interest in recouping the millions of dollars and years of research that they have invested in a particular medicine. This inherent conflict of interest should be obvious. In addition, many medicines are being used for conditions other than what the FDA approved

> **Natural approaches help resolve the underlying problem causing the pain.**

them for. The terrifying aspect of this is that there may be only minimal or limited collaborating clinical research and evidence that validates these medicines for non-FDA approved clinical uses.

I have grave concerns when the established medical community, with their history of oppression of natural approaches, and use of medications and procedures which are invalid by their own standards, are demanding an account of alternative medicine. Make no mistake, I do believe in the need for clinical research demonstrating the virtues of alternative medicine, but it also needs to be performed by those who do not have their own bias and agendas to carry it out.

The good news is that research and clinical studies are being carried out, with a major increase taking place here in the United States. We have even formed a government bureaucracy to regulate and institute policies for alternative medicine, The Office of Alternative Medicine (OAM) which is a part of the National Institute of Health (NIH). Regardless of the political and scientific ramifications, natural approaches are being used by millions of Americans on a day-to-day basis, many with excellent results, and that number is growing each day.

Natural approaches to pain relief are many and varied. There are natural substances which can directly impact and relieve pain. Examples of these would be DLPA (DL-phenylalanine, an amino acid), glucosamine sulfate, feverfew and white willow bark (herbs). Perhaps even more importantly is the use of natural approaches and substances to resolve underlying conditions which create and cause pain. The first thing to decipher is what the condition is that may be causing the problem and pain. In some cases, this will be obvious; especially if the cause is from injury or trauma to some part of us.

Take a look at this example of a natural approach to injury. Some of the approaches listed in the example you have certainly heard before. While many of you consider it common knowledge to apply ice to an injured area; very few of you may recognize this approach as a "natural" therapy.

As you can see from this scenario, this natural approach provides complete care for an injury to the knee, including direct and indirect pain relief.

Example of a Natural Approach to Injury

You hurt your right knee as a result from falling onto the knee after tripping over a curb. There is pain in the right knee, a scrape to the skin with a bruise over the kneecap and mild swelling, all from the impact of the right knee with the pavement.

1. Clean the knee and surrounding tissue with witch hazel liquid (an antiseptic) to remove debris and blood.

2. Inspect the knee for damage.

3. If there is mild or moderate bruising and/or swelling...
    A. Apply ice to the knee and keep it elevated.
    B. Remove the ice, and apply calendula gel and arnica gel to the knee to speed healing, reduce pain, bruising and swelling.

---

4. If the swelling is profound...

A. Wrap the knee in an ace bandage to apply compression and support to the knee.

B. Take white willow bark and bromelain orally, two capsules 2-3 times per day for pain control and as an anti-inflammatory. If you have a stomach condition such as an ulcer or chronic gastritis, an alternate natural substance may be needed.

C. During the initial 24 to 48 hours, limit your activities, rest the knee and keep it elevated as much as possible.

If this injury is only a simple contusion or mild sprain/strain to the knee, it will heal itself within a few days.

If the pain and other symptoms do not resolve within 4-7 days, you will need to follow up with a health care professional for evaluation of the knee to assess further damage.

But what of other, more serious conditions? Can natural approaches help resolve pain syndromes involved with chronic disease? In many cases the answer is yes.

Lets look at the disease process arthritis. Arthritis literally means "inflamed joints" and there are many different forms it can take. Included in this group is Osteoarthritis, Rheumatoid Arthritis, Juvenile Rheumatoid Arthritis, Ankylosing Spondylitis, Reiter's Syndrome, Psoriatic Arthritis, Lyme Disease Arthritis, Infectious and Bacterial Arthritis to name a few.

Lets look specifically at Osteoarthritis (OA), the most prevalent arthritic form. It is an age-related, chronic, degenerative joint disease that is specific to the joints of the body. This means that as we age, there will be progressive degeneration and deterioration of our joints. Generally, this occurs gradually over the years but may occur earlier in life due to traumas, injuries, genetic factors and other reasons. There are many mitigating factors to this degeneration, including those just mentioned and factors such as overall health, diet, exercise, whether a person has a history of smoking, etc. All of these factors will effect the amount and speed of the degenerative processes in the joints. This translates into each individual having their own levels of joint degeneration which may vary greatly from others within the same age group. However, the fact remains that this is an age related degeneration and will occur regardless of other factors.

Osteoarthritis is commonly found in many joints of the body including the spine, hips, knees, ankles and feet, shoulders, elbows, wrist, hands and fingers. Typically the pain associated with osteoarthritis is of a dull, aching nature that is within and/or around the joint. Depending on the level of pain and degeneration within a particular joint, there can be other associated signs and symptoms. These include such things as reduced, limited, altered or restricted range of joint motion, joint stiffness, crackling and popping of the joint (called Crepitus), bony changes within the joint (bony overgrowth, bone spurs, etc.), and altered usage and muscle tone around an affected joint because of pain and these other symptoms. The impact of osteoarthritis is staggering, both in terms of its debilitating effects on older people and its tremendous cost medically. Usage of over-the-counter and prescriptions pain medications as treatment of osteoarthritis is common in traditional medicine. But is there a better

Natural Approaches for Osteoarthritis

Vitamins:
Vitamin A, beta carotene, Vitamin C, Vitamin E, all the B-vitamins, especially B3 (niacin), B5 (pantothenic acid), B6 (pyridoxine), B12 (cobalamin), Folic acid, and Vitamin K.

Minerals and Trace Elements:
Calcium, magnesium, copper, zinc, silica, boron, manganese, and selenium.

Enzymes: (proteolytic and digestive)
Bromelain, pancreatin, amylase, lactase, lipase, papain, pepsin, betaine HCl, and protease.

Other Supplements:
Glucosamine sulfate, chondroitin sulfate, MSM, NAG (N-acetylglucosamine), SOD (Superoxide dismutase), coenzyme Q-10, DMG (Dimethylglycine), bioflavonoids, germanium, pycogenol, grape seed extract, DL-Phenylalanine (DLPA), L-cysteine, shark cartilage, sea cucumber, primrose oil, fish oil, flaxseed oil, borage oil, etc.

Herbs:
Alfalfa, garlic, cat's claw, feverfew, ginger, cayenne (capsicum), wintergreen, white willow bark, white oak bark, boswellia, brigham, burdock root, celery seed, corn silk, devil's claw, horsetail, nettle, parsley, yucca, etc.

way to treat this malady? Absolutely!

There are many natural approaches to osteoarthritis, some which have been used for literally centuries, while others have only become available recently. Many of these, especially the vitamins, minerals, trace elements, enzymes and other supplements, provide overall nutrient needs for general health while also impacting osteoarthritis both directly and indirectly. The previous page features is a brief list of those nutrient substances and herbs that can provide relief for osteoarthritis. See Section Three for more detailed information.

You can see from the number of substances listed that there are many different nutrients and herbs which are known to have a positive impact on osteoarthritis and our joints in general. The key to utilizing these natural substances and alternative approaches is using them in therapeutic doses and matching the specific substances with your individual needs and complaints. While these substances can generally be used safely by the public, it is always a good idea to be evaluated by a health care professional; especially one who is trained in natural approaches and can set up and monitor a natural-based protocol for you.

These are some examples of how natural approaches and alternative medicine can be used to attack our pain and the underlying conditions which cause our aches and pains. In reviewing this material, it must be made clear that treating pain from natural approaches almost always addresses the underlying condition. This is a critical concept and must be understood!

Many people become discouraged when they are unable to manage their pain relief using natural methods. When I review their approach, I typically find a group of common mistakes.

- The first mistake is that they have not been using either the right substances or the correct combination of substances.

- The second mistake is not taking the substances in doses which will elicit a therapeutic response. This is very important and must be approached with caution, under the guidance of a health care professional.

- A third mistake is very common and is usually caused because of a misunderstanding of the time required to get both pain relief and a positive impact on the disease or condition. I have found that many people stop taking the natural substances before they can penetrate their biochemical systems and adequately elicit a response. Unfortunately, this is a difficult problem to overcome because we have been indoctrinated in the concept of "immediate pain relief," typically by taking an over-the-counter or prescription pain medication.

There are definitely natural substances which can provide immediate pain relief. However, these are most often used with other substances that will address the resolution of the underlying condition. This important concept, as I have previously stated, it is critical for any long term pain relief. With this in mind, lets look at the other ways we seek to achieve pain relief.

Standard and Non-Standard Approaches to Natural Pain Relief

Pain relief can be simple or very difficult, regardless of how you approach it. From a natural-based perspective, this may appear very confusing. I suspect this is based more on the lack of knowledge in regard to natural approaches, their proper use and implementation, rather than any specific failing with them in general.

To understand how natural approaches can be utilized, one must first learn what they are capable of and how they may be used. As previously discussed, pain relief can be achieved in two main ways.

● Address the pain directly with particular substances and therapeutic interventions.

● Resolve the underlying disease or condition; thus creating pain relief from this resolution.

But how does alternative medicine address this second issue? As you have seen from the example in regard to Osteoarthritis, natural approaches work to address a variety of underlying components that are part and parcel of a particular condition. This can include any or all of the following:

Improve, repair, rebuild, and **rejuvenate** the various systems of the body including the:
- Gastrointestinal/digestive system
- Circulatory system
- Endocrine/hormonal system

- Metabolic system
- Nervous system
- Muscular and skeletal system

As part of your recovery you will also need to:

- Reduce inflammation
- Eliminate food allergies and hypersensitivities
- Normalize weight problems
- Correct nutritional deficiencies (both clinical and subclinical)
- Alter poor whole food dietary habits, etc.

It is important to attack the problem from many directions at the same time. This can prove to be extremely valuable, since most diseases and conditions effect many different systems of the body.

Lets take this a step further. To resolve a particular condition you must address any and all aspects and effects created by that entity. Ignoring or bypassing one or more components may eliminate any real chance at resolving that condition.

When I set up my natural-based protocols, I always review the impact on the different systems of the body and set up the natural interventions based on that knowledge. A positive outcome is the goal, whether that is through decreasing the patient's symptoms, improving functionality and quality of life, or the complete resolution of the disease or condition.

To resolve a particular condition you must address any and all aspects and effects of that condition.

Module One:

Natural Pain Relieving Substances

Module One presents a number of natural substances that can be used for pain relief and/or that can be used to resolve underlying conditions. The information contained herein is presented under the following headings: Vitamins, Minerals, Other Supplements and Substances, Enzymes, Amino Acids, Herbals Homeopathics, and Topical Approaches Each of these categories will include those substances that are pertinent to resolving pain relief. The substances listed here are for oral and topical applications.

When we evaluate these various substances for there uses in natural approaches, especially in regard to the vitamins, minerals, other supplements and substances, and enzymes, it must be recognized that each of these substances plays an integral role in human nutrition. This means that they are a necessary part of normal health and thus can, and usually are, negatively effected by many conditions. I bring this up because it could be said that each of these substances may have an impact on pain relief, especially in an indirect manner. I have focused on those substances which are known to have specific ties to relieving pain. Please remember that each of these listed substances may have general effects on pain relief or may effect particular conditions.

Vitamins

Vitamin C

Vitamin C is an incredible nutrient. It has many important qualities. Vitamin C is a water-soluble vitamin and is essential in human nutrition. Vitamin C is used extensively in the United States and is very popular. One of its primary roles and functions is in the formation of collagen, the main protein connective tissue substance in the body. Collagen is critical for the growth and repair of body tissue and cells. It is very important for healthy gums, blood vessels, bones, and teeth. Vitamin C also plays an important role as one of the primary antioxidants in the body countering the negative destructive effects of free radicals.

Vitamin C does many things within the body: It increases the absorption of iron and is needed for the metabolism of folic acid, tyrosine, and phenylalanine. It can help prevent cancer, protects against infection, enhance immunity, aid in the production of anti-stress hormones and protect us against the harmful effects of pollution and cigarette smoke.

Vitamin C is very important in a number of disease processes including atherosclerosis and high blood pressure. It can decrease cholesterol levels.

Vitamin C promotes healing within the body, especially in the healing of wounds and burns, also in healing after surgery. Vitamin C protects against blood clotting and bruising as it reduces capillary fragility. It plays a role in the manufacture of certain nerve transmitters and hormones, especially in the production of anti-stress hormones. Vitamin C strengthens the immune system and aids in the prevention of many types of viral and bacterial infections. It also acts as a natural laxative, lowers the incidence of blood clots in the veins, reduces the effects of many allergy-producing substances, extends life by enabling protein cells to hold together and can reduce the risk of cataracts.

Vitamin C's actions are very impressive as a singular substance. Vitamin C works with and reinforces other antioxidants, especially Vitamin E. These two vitamins increase the actions of each other, thus having a greater effect on their antioxidant activity on free radicals.

The human body cannot manufacture Vitamin C. Because of this, it must be obtained daily from our diets or from supplementation. There is a lot of controversy in regard to the optimal amounts of Vitamin C necessary for general health needs and in the treatment of disease processes. This controversy has been going on for a number of years and it does not look like it will be resolved anytime soon. As an example, with serious diseases, such as Cancer, very large amounts of Vitamin C may be necessary as part of a natural protocol. However, many within the medical community would dispute this approach.

Scurvy is a disease caused by Vitamin C deficiency. It is characterized by poor wound healing, soft and spongy bleeding gums, edema, extreme weakness, and "pinpoint" hemorrhages under the skin. More common signs of lesser degrees of deficiency, including gums that bleed when brushed, increased susceptibility to infection, especially colds and bronchial infections, joint pains, lack of energy, poor digestion, prolonged healing time, a tendency to bruise easily, and tooth loss.

Sources: Vitamin C is found in a large variety of fruits and vegetables. Good sources include asparagus, avocados, beet greens, black currants, broccoli, brussels sprouts, cantaloupe, collards, dandelion greens, grapefruit, lemons, mangos, mustard greens, onions, oranges, papayas, green peas, sweet peppers, pineapple, rose hips, spinach, strawberries, tomatoes and watercress.

A number of herbs also contain Vitamin C. Included in this group are alfalfa, burdock root, cayenne, chickweed, eyebright, fennel seed, fenugreek, hops, horsetail, kelp, peppermint, mullein, nettle, oat straw, parsley, plantain, raspberry leaf, red clover, rose hips, skullcap, yarrow and yellow dock.

There are many major conditions where Vitamin C is of value. Please note that I have underlined some of the disorders which have pain syndromes related to them: Asthma, allergies, atherosclerosis, <u>autoimmune disorders,</u> <u>backache,</u> <u>cancer</u> and chemotherapy support, candidiasis, capillary fragility, cataracts, cervical dysplasia, Crohn's disease, <u>common cold,</u> coronary artery disease, diabetes, eczema, fatigue, <u>gallbladder disease</u>, gingivitis, glaucoma, hay fever, <u>hepatitis</u>, herpes simplex, <u>herpes zoster</u>, high blood pressure, high cholesterol, hives, immune function, infections, infertility, iron deficiency, macular degeneration, menopause, menorrhagia (heavy menstruation), mitral valve prolapse, morning sickness, multiple sclerosis, <u>osteoarthritis,</u> Parkinson's disease, periodontal disease, peptic ulcers, peripheral vascular disease, preeclampsia, <u>recurrent ear infection,</u> <u>rheumatoid</u> <u>arthritis,</u> skin ulcers, <u>sports injuries,</u> urinary tract infections, wound healing and vitilego.

Ascorbic Acid is <u>NOT</u> the Best Form of C - Mineral Ascorbates are Preferred!

Many people are under the false impression that Vitamin C is ascorbic acid. In truth, this is just one form of Vitamin C and it is not the form I recommend. Ascorbic acid is highly acidic (pH of 2 or 3) and can disrupt the sensitive pH of the body. The pH of the urine is lowered which is increasingly irritating to the kidneys and bladder, inducing a strong diuretic action, which results in a marked loss of valuable mineral from the body, and can cause diarrhea, flatulence, nausea, heartburn, stomach irritation, and can possibly lead to or irritate ulcers.

I prefer Vitamin C in the form of mineral ascorbates (calcium ascorbate, potassium ascorbate, magnesium ascorbate, etc.) which are pH neutral. This is the form of Vitamin C produced in animals who do manufacture their own Vitamin C. Only humans, the guinea pig, the monkey, the ape, and a type of bat cannot manufacture mineral ascorbates in the body. Mineral ascorbates are highly absorbable by our cells and therefore much more beneficial.

Precautions: There are many substances which can deplete Vitamin C in the body including alcohol, analgesics, antidepressants, anticoagulants, oral contraceptives, steroids and smoking. An important caution needs to be addressed when taking aspirin and Vitamin C in the form of ascorbic acid, especially in large doses, can cause side effects such as listed above. (Lytle, Hanck, Creagan, Gupte, Werbach)

Vitamin B-1

Vitamin B1, called Thiamine, is a water-soluble vitamin. Thiamine enhances circulation and assists in blood formation, carbohydrate metabolism, and the production of hydrochloric acid, which is important for proper digestion. Thiamine, also optimizes cognitive activity, brain function and its impact on mental attitude. It has a positive effect on energy production, growth, normal appetite, and learning capacity, and is needed for muscle tone of the intestines, stomach, and heart.

In general, B1 keeps the nervous system, muscles and heart functioning normally. Thiamine also acts as an antioxidant, protecting the body from the degenerative effects of aging, alcohol consumption, and smoking. It has mild diuretic effects. Thiamine can help fight air and seasickness. It can help relieve dental postoperative pain and aid in the treatment of herpes zoster. Thiamine can mimic the important neurotransmitter involved in memory, acetylcholine. As with all B vitamins, Thiamine is intricately involved with other B-vitamins in energy metabolism. Magnesium is required in the conversion of Thiamine to its active form.

Beriberi, a nervous system disease, is caused by a deficiency of Thiamine. In true deficiency, the symptoms can include mental confusion (and in severe cases, psychosis), muscle wasting, fluid retention high blood pressure, difficulty walking and heart disturbances. Other symptoms resulting from thiamine deficiency include constipation, edema, enlarged liver, fatigue, forgetfulness, gastrointestinal disturbances, heart changes, irritability, labored breathing loss of appetite, muscle atrophy, nervousness, numbness of the hands and feet, pain and sensitivity, poor coordination, tingling sensations, weak and sore muscles, general weakness, and severe weight loss.

Sources: The richest food sources of Thiamine include brown rice, egg yolks, fish, legumes, liver, peanuts, peas, pork, poultry, rice bran, wheat germ, and whole grains. Other sources are asparagus, brewer's yeast, broccoli, brussels sprouts, kelp, most nuts, oatmeal, plums, dried prunes, raisins, spirulina and watercress. Herbs that contain thiamine include alfalfa, bladderwrack, burdock root, catnip, cayenne, chamomile, chickweed, eyebright, fennel seed fenugreek, hops, nettle, oat straw, parsley, peppermint, raspberry leaf, red clover, rose hips, sage, yarrow and yellow dock.

The principal use of Thiamine is to prevent thiamin deficiency, especially in diabetes, Crohn's disease, multiple sclerosis, and other neurological diseases and to prevent and treat impaired mental function in the elderly, in Alzheimer's patients, and in epileptics being treat with Dilantin.

Conditions that Vitamin B1 can be used to treat and are supportive include AIDS, alcoholism, anemia, cancer, canker sores (mouth ulcers), Crohn's disease, diabetes mellitus, epilepsy, fibromyalgia, glaucoma, multiple sclerosis, neuralgia and neuropathy, pain, Parkinson's disease, pregnancy-related illness and support, rheumatism and wound healing.

Precautions: There are different medications which can decrease the levels of thiamine in the body. These include antibiotics, sulfa drugs and oral contraceptives. (Lenot, Mazzoni, Quirin, Charonnat, Werbach)

Vitamin B-6

Vitamin B6, called Pyridoxine, is involved in more bodily functions than almost any other single nutrient. It is an extremely important B vitamin involved in the formation of body proteins and structural compounds, chemical transmitters in the nervous system, red blood cells, and prostaglandins. Vitamin B6 is also critical in maintaining hormonal balance and proper immune function. It affects both physical and mental health. It is beneficial if you suffer from water retention, and is necessary for the production of hydrochloric acid and the absorption of fats and protein.

Pyridoxine also aids in maintaining sodium and potassium balance, and promotes red blood cell formation. It is required by the nervous system, and is needed for normal brain function and for the synthesis of the nucleic acids RNA and DNA, which contain the genetic instructions for the reproduction of all cells and for normal cellular growth. It activates many enzymes and aids in the absorption of Vitamin B12, in immune system function, and in antibody production. Pyridoxine is required for the proper functioning of more than 60 different enzymes. It plays a vital role in the multiplication of all cells and is, therefore, of critical importance to a healthy pregnancy and proper functioning immune system, mucous membrane, skin and red blood cells.

Vitamin B6 plays a role in cancer immunity and aids in the prevention of arteriosclerosis. It inhibits the formation of a toxic chemical called homocysteine, which attacks the heart muscle and allows the deposition of cholesterol around the heart muscle. Pyridoxine acts a mild diuretic, reducing the symptoms of premenstrual syndrome, and it may be useful in preventing oxalate kidney stones, as well. It is helpful in the treatment of allergies, arthritis, and asthma.

A deficiency of Vitamin B6 may be recognized by anemia, convulsions, depression, glucose intolerance, impaired nerve function, eczema or seborrhea, headaches, nausea, flaky skin, a sore tongue, and vomiting. Other possible signs of deficiency include acne, anorexia, arthritis, conjunctivitis, cracks or sores on the mouth and lips, depression, dizziness, fatigue, hyperirritability, impaired wound healing, inflammation of the mouth and gums, learning difficulties, weak memory, hair loss, hearing problems, numbness, oily facial skin, stunted growth, and tingling sensations. Carpal tunnel syndrome has been linked to a deficiency of Vitamin B6 as well. Lack of Vitamin B6 greatly affects pregnancy and plays a critical role in brain chemistry because it is involved in the manufacture of all amino acid neurotransmitters (e.g., serotonin, dopamine, melatonin, epinephrine, norepinephrine, etc.)

Sources: Almost all foods contain some Vitamin B6, however, the following foods have the highest amounts: brewer's yeast, carrots, chicken, eggs, fish, meat, peas, spinach, sunflower seeds, walnuts, and wheat germ. Other sources include avocado, bananas, beans, blackstrap molasses, broccoli, brown rice and other whole grains, cabbage, cantaloupe, corn, plantains, potatoes, rice bran, and soybeans. Herbs that contain B6 include alfalfa, catnip and oat straw.

Vitamin B6 is one of the most utilized and valued nutritional supplements. It in fact plays an important role in over 100 conditions. The most common conditions that Vitamin B6 impacts are: Asthma, atherosclerosis, autism, canker sores, cardiovascular disease, carpal tunnel syndrome, chemotherapy support, depression, diabetes (prevention and diabetic complications), epilepsy, fibrocystic breast disease, high cholesterol, immune enhancement, kidney stones, morning sickness (from pregnancy), osteoporosis, and premenstrual syndrome.

Precautions: Vitamin B6 should not be taken by any person taking levodopa for treatment of Parkinson's Disease. (Bernstein, Werbach)

Vitamin B-12

Vitamin B12, called Cyanocobalamin or cobalamin, is another water-soluble vitamin. It is needed to prevent anemia, by regulating the formation and regeneration of red blood cells. It helps in the utilization of iron. This vitamin is also required for proper digestion, absorption of foods, the synthesis of protein, and the proper metabolism of carbohydrates and fats. It aids in cell formation and cellular longevity. In addition, Vitamin B12 prevents nerve damage, maintains fertility, and promotes normal growth and development by maintaining the fatty sheaths that cover and protect nerve endings. Vitamin B12 is linked to the production of acetylcholine, a neurotransmitter that assists memory and learning. It needs to be combined with calcium during absorption to properly benefit the body. Vitamin B12 promotes growth and increased appetite in children, increases energy, relieve irritability, improve concentration, memory and balance.

Vitamin B12 works well with folic acid in many body processes, including the synthesis of DNA, red blood cells and the myelin sheath that surrounds nerve cells and speeds the conduction of the signals along nerve cells.

A Vitamin B12 deficiency can be caused by malabsorption, which is most common in elderly people and in those with digestive disorders. The main deficiency of Vitamin B12 is Pernicious anemia. Other deficiency symptoms can include an abnormal gait, chronic fatigue, constipation, depression, digestive disorders, dizziness, drowsiness, enlargement of the liver, eye disorders, hallucinations, headaches, inflammation of the tongue, irritability, labored breathing, memory loss, moodiness, nervousness, neurological damage, numbness, palpitations, pernicious anemia, pins and needles sensations, ringing in the ears, and spinal cord degeneration. Usually, a deficiency of Vitamin B12 affects the brain and nervous system first.

Strict vegetarians must remember that they require Vitamin B12 supplementation, as the vitamin is found almost exclusively in animal tissue. Although people adopting a strict vegetarian diet may not see signs of the deficiency for some time as the body can store up to five years worth of Vitamin B12, deficiency signs will eventually develop.

Sources: Vitamin B12 is found in all foods of animal origin. The largest amounts of Vitamin B12 are found in brewer's yeast, clams, eggs, herring, kidney, liver, mackerel, milk and dairy products and seafood. While Vitamin B12 is not found in many vegetables; it is available from sea vegetables, such as dulse, kelp, kombu, nori, and from soybeans and soy products. It is also present in the herbs, alfalfa, bladderwrack and hops.

Vitamin B12's uses are appropriate for many conditions. These include Aids, Alzheimer's disease, asthma, atherosclerosis, bursitis, Crohn's disease, depression, diabetes and diabetic neuropathy, high cholesterol, impaired mental function in the elderly, infertility, multiple sclerosis, osteoporosis, pernicious anemia, tinnitus, and vitilego.

Precautions: Anticoagulants and anti-gout medications may inhibit absorption of Vitamin B12. (Hanck, Hieber, Dettori, Bruggemann, Werbach)

Vitamin E

Vitamin E is a fat-soluble vitamin and is an antioxidant that is important in the prevention of cancer and cardiovascular disease. It improves circulation, is necessary for tissue repair, and is useful in treating premenstrual syndrome and fibrocystic disease of the breast. It promotes normal blood clotting and healing, reduces scarring from some wounds, reduces blood pressure, aids in preventing cataracts, improves athletic performance, and relaxes leg cramps. It also maintains healthy nerves and muscles while strengthening capillary walls. In addition, it promotes healthy skin and hair, and helps to prevent anemia and retrolental fibroplasia, an eye disorder that can affect premature infants. It is very important to immune function, especially in providing protection during times of stress and chronic viral illness. Vitamin E helps retards cellular aging due to oxidation, supplies oxygen to the body to give more endurance, protects the lungs against air pollution by working with Vitamin A. It can alleviate fatigue, prevent thick scar formation externally, accelerate healing of burns, lower blood pressure and help alleviate leg cramps.

As an antioxidant, Vitamin E prevents cell damage by inhibiting the oxidation of lipids (fats) and the formation of free radicals. It protects other fat-soluble vitamins from destruction by oxygen, and aids in the utilization of Vitamin A and protects it from destruction oxygen. It retards aging and may prevent age spots as well. Vitamin E is also important for healthy reproductive systems in both men and women.

Vitamin E deficiency may result in damage to red blood cells and destruction of nerves. Signs of deficiency can include infertility, menstrual problems, muscular weakness, neuromuscular impairment, poor coordination, shortened red blood cell life span and breaking of red blood cells, spontaneous abortion (miscarriage) and uterine degeneration. Low levels of Vitamin E in the body have been linked to both bowel cancer and breast cancer. Epidemiological links have been identified between the increase in the incidence of heart disease and the increasing lack of Vitamin E in the diet due to our reliance on over-processed foods.

Vitamin E is actually a family of eight different but related molecules that fall into two major groups: the tocopherols and tocotrienols. Within each group, there are alpha, beta, gamma, and delta forms. Of all eight of these molecules, it is the alpha-tocopherol form that is the most potent.

Sources: Vitamin E is found in the following food sources: cold-pressed vegetable oils, dark green leafy vegetables, legumes, nuts, seeds, and whole grains. Significant quantities of this vitamin are also found in brown rice, cornmeal, dulse, eggs, kelp, desiccated liver, milk, oatmeal, organ meats, soybeans, sweet potatoes, watercress, wheat, and wheat germ. Herbs that contain Vitamin E include alfalfa, bladderwrack, dandelion, dong quai, flaxseed, nettle, oat straw, raspberry leaf, and rose hips.

The principal use of Vitamin E is as an antioxidant. Through this function, it provides protection against heart disease, cancer and strokes. Vitamin E supplementation is useful in a long list of health conditions, including AIDS, alcohol-induced liver disease, allergy, anemia, angina, arrhythmias, atherosclerosis, autoimmune disorders, cancer, capillary fragility, cardiomyopathy, cataract, cervical dysplasia, diabetes, dysmenorrhea, eczema, epilepsy, fibrocystic breast disease, fibromyalgia, gallstones, hepatitis, herpes simplex and zoster, immunodepression, infections, inflammation, intermittent claudication, lupus, macular degeneration, menopausal symptoms, multiple sclerosis, myopathy, neuralgia, neuromuscular degeneration, osteoarthritis, Parkinson's disease, peptic ulcers, periodontal disease, peripheral vascular disease, pregnancy, premenstrual syndrome, Raynauds, disease, rheumatoid arthritis, scleroderma, seborrheic dermatitis, skin ulcers, ulcerative colitis and wound healing.

Precautions: If you have been diagnosed with diabetes, rheumatic heart disease or an overactive thyroid conditions, do not take more than doses recommended by your health care professional. With blood thinning medications do not take more than 1200 IU per day. (Kryzhacovskii, Werbach)

Vitamin K

Vitamin K is needed for the production of prothrombin, which is necessary for blood clotting. It is also essential for bone formation and repair; it is necessary for the synthesis of osteocalcin, the protein I bone tissue on which calcium crystallizes. Consequently, it may help prevent osteoporosis.

Vitamin K plays an important role in the intestines and aids in converting glucose into glycogen for storage in the liver, promoting healthy liver function. It may increase resistance to infection in children and help prevent cancers that target the inner linings of the organs. It aids in promoting longevity.

A deficiency of this vitamin can cause abnormal and/or internal bleeding.

Vitamin K exists in three forms. Vitamin K1 and K2 occur naturally; Vitamin K3 is synthetic.

Sources: Vitamin K is found in some foods, including asparagus, blackstrap molasses, broccoli, brussels sprouts, cabbage, cauliflower, dark green leafy vegetables, egg yolks, liver, oatmeal, oats, rye, safflower oil, soybeans, and wheat. Herbs that can supply Vitamin K include alfalfa, green tea, kelp, nettle, oat straw, and shepherd's purse.

The majority of the body's supply of this vitamin is synthesized by the "friendly" bacteria normally present in the intestines.

Precautions: Antibiotics increase the need for dietary or supplemental Vitamin K. Antibiotics, which kill both "friendly" and "bad" bacteria, interferes with Vitamin K production in the body. Large doses of synthetic Vitamin K taken during the last few weeks of pregnancy can result in a toxic reaction in the newborn. (Hanck, Werbach)

Minerals

Calcium

Calcium is vital for the formation of strong bones and teeth and for the maintenance of healthy gums. It is also important in the maintenance of a regular heartbeat and the transmission of nerve impulses. Calcium lowers cholesterol levels and helps prevent cardiovascular disease. It is needed for muscular growth and contraction, and for the prevention of muscle cramps. It may increase the rate of bone growth and bone mineral density in children and adults. This important mineral is also essential in blood clotting and helps prevent cancer. It may lower blood pressure and prevent bone loss associated with osteoporosis as well. Calcium provides energy and participates in the protein structuring of RNA and DNA. It is also involved in the activation of several enzymes, including lipase, which breaks down fats for utilization by the body. In addition, calcium maintains proper cell membrane permeability, aids in neuromuscular activity, helps to keep the skin healthy, and protects against the development of pre-eclampsia during pregnancy.

Calcium protects the bones and teeth from lead by inhibiting absorption of this toxic metal. If there is a calcium deficiency, lead can be absorbed by the body and deposited in the teeth and bones.

Calcium deficiency can lead to: Aching joints, brittle nails, eczema, elevated blood cholesterol, heart palpitations, hypertension, insomnia, muscle cramps, nervousness, numbness in the arms and/or legs, a pasty complexion, rheumatoid arthritis, rickets, and tooth decay. Deficiencies of calcium are also associated with cognitive impairment, convulsions, depression, delusions and hyperactivity.

Sources: Calcium is found in milk and dairy foods, salmon, sardines, seafood, and green leafy vegetables. Food sources include almonds, asparagus, blackstrap molasses, brewer's yeast, broccoli, buttermilk, cabbage, carob, cheese, collards, dandelion greens, dulse, figs, goat's milk, kelp, mustard greens, oats, prunes, sesame seeds, soybeans, tofu, watercress, and yogurt.

Herbs that contain calcium include alfalfa, burdock root, cayenne, chamomile, chickweed, chicory, dandelion, eyebright, fennel seed, fenugreek, flaxseed, hops, horsetail, kelp, lemongrass, mullein, nettle, oat straw, parsley, peppermint, plantain, raspberry leaves, red clover, rose hips, yarrow and yellow dock.

Heavy exercise can hinder calcium uptake while moderate exercise promotes it. Female athletes and menopausal women need greater amounts of calcium than other women because their estrogen levels are lower. Taking calcium with iron reduces the effect of both minerals.

Precautions: Calcium may interfere with the effects of verapamil, a calcium channel blocker prescribed for heart problems and high blood pressure. Calcium supplements should not be taken by persons with a history of kidney stones or kidney disease.

Magnesium

Magnesium is a vital catalyst in enzyme activity, especially the activity of those enzymes involved in energy production. It assists in calcium and potassium uptake. A deficiency of magnesium interferes with the transmission of nerve and muscle impulses, causing irritability and nervousness. Magnesium supplementation can help prevent depression, dizziness, muscle weakness and twitching, PMS, and also aid in maintaining the body's proper pH balance.

Magnesium is necessary to prevent the calcification of soft tissue. This essential mineral protects the arterial linings from stress caused by sudden blood pressure changes, and plays a role in the formation of bone and in carbohydrate and mineral metabolism. With Vitamin B6, magnesium helps to reduce and dissolve calcium phosphate kidney stones. Recent research has shown that magnesium may help prevent cardiovascular disease, osteoporosis, and certain forms of cancer, and it may reduce cholesterol levels. It is effective in preventing premature labor and convulsions in pregnant women. Magnesium combined with Vitamin B6 may prevent calcium oxalate kidney stones.

Magnesium deficiency includes confusion, insomnia, irritability, poor digestion, rapid heartbeat, seizures, and tantrums. Often, a magnesium deficiency can be synonymous with diabetes. It is considered that magnesium deficiency are at the root of many cardiovascular problems. It may cause fatal cardiac arrhythmia, hypertension, and sudden cardiac arrest, as well as asthma, chronic fatigue, chronic pain syndromes, depression, insomnia, irritable bowel syndrome, and pulmonary disorders.

Sources: Magnesium is found in most foods, especially dairy products, fish, meat, and seafood. Food sources which have magnesium include apples, apricots, avocados, bananas, blackstrap molasses, brewer's yeast, brown rice, cantaloupe, dulse, figs, garlic, grapefruit, green leafy vegetables, kelp, lemons, lima beans, millet, nuts, peaches, black-eyed peas, salmon, sesame seeds, soybeans, tofu, watercress, wheat, and whole grains. Herbs that contain magnesium include alfalfa, bladderwrack, catnip, cayenne, chamomile, chickweed, dandelion, eyebright, fennel seed, fenugreek, hops, horsetail, lemongrass, licorice, mullein, nettle, oat straw parsley, peppermint, raspberry leaf, red clover, sage, yarrow and yellow dock.

Precautions: Alcohol and diuretics can decrease the levels of magnesium.

Copper

Copper has many functions. It aids in the formation of bone, hemoglobin, red blood cells, and works in balance with zinc and Vitamin C to form elastin. It is involved in the healing process, energy production, hair and skin coloring, and taste sensitivity. This mineral is also needed for healthy nerves and joints.

An early sign of copper deficiency is osteoporosis. Copper is essential for the formation of collagen, one of the fundamental proteins making up bones, skin, and connective tissue. Other possible signs of copper deficiency include anemia, baldness, diarrhea, general weakness, impaired respiratory function, and skin sores. A lack of copper can also lead to increased blood fat levels.

Sources: Copper is found in cookware and plumbing. Copper is found in many foods including almonds, avocados, barley, beans, beets, blackstrap molasses, broccoli, garlic, lentils, liver, mushrooms, nuts, oats, oranges, pecans, radishes, raisins, salmon, seafood, soybeans, and green leafy vegetables.

Precautions: Excessive intake of copper can lead to toxicity, which has been associated with depression, irritability, nausea and vomiting, nervousness, and joint and muscle pain. (Bhathene, Werbach)

Selenium

Selenium's principal function is to inhibit the oxidation of fats. It is a vital antioxidant, especially when combined with Vitamin E. It protects the immune system by preventing the formation of free radicals, which can damage the body. It has also been found to function as a preventive against the formation of certain types of tumors. Selenium and Vitamin E act synergistically to aid in the production of antibodies and to help maintain a healthy heart and liver. This trace element is needed form pancreatic function and tissue elasticity. When combined with Vitamin E and zinc, it may also provide relief from an enlarged prostate. Selenium supplementation has been found to protect the liver in people with alcoholic cirrhosis.

Selenium deficiency has been linked to cancer and heart disease. It has also been associated with exhaustion, growth impairment, high cholesterol levels, infections, liver impairment, pancreatic insufficiency, and sterility.

Sources: Selenium can be found in meat and grains, depending on the selenium content of the soil where the food is raised. It can be found in brazil nuts, brewer's yeast, broccoli, brown rice, chicken, diary products, dulse, garlic, kelp, liver, molasses, onions, salmon, seafood, yeast, tuna, vegetables, wheat germ and whole grains. Herbs that contain selenium include alfalfa, burdock root, catnip, cayenne, chamomile, chickweed, fennel seed, fenugreek, garlic, ginseng, hawthorn berry, hops, horsetail, lemongrass, milk thistle nettle, oat straw, parsley, peppermint, raspberry leaf, rose hips, uva ursi, yarrow, and yellow dock.

Precautions: Excessive selenium levels can cause arthritis, brittle nails, "garlic-like" breath, gastrointestinal disorders, hair loss, irritability, liver and kidney impairment, a metallic taste in the mouth, pallor, skin eruptions, and yellowish skin. (Van Rij, Jameson, Werbach)

Germanium

Germanium improves cellular and tissue oxygenation. Germanium is a powerful antioxidant that increases cell respiration, dramatically improves aerobic performance and may also protect against hypoxia and respiratory distress. Germanium is useful against allergies, colds, flu, cold sores, hepatitis, and other liver problems and is a powerful immune system stimulant with anti-bacterial and anti-viral effects. It helps to fight pain, keep the immune system functioning properly, and rid the body of toxins and poisons. Researchers have shown that consuming foods containing organic germanium is an effective way to increase tissue oxygenation, because, the hemoglobin, germanium acts as a carrier of oxygen to the cells. A Japanese scientist, Kazuhiko Asai, found that an intake of 100 to 300 mg of germanium per day improved many illnesses, including rheumatoid arthritis, food allergies, elevated cholesterol, candidiasis, chronic viral infections, cancer, and AIDS.

Studies suggest that when administered daily, germanium is effective against free radical pathology, lipid peroxidation, and degenerative diseases. It is also useful in fighting heavy metal poisoning.

Sources: The following foods contain germanium include garlic, shiitake mushrooms, onions, and the herbs aloe vera, comfrey, ginseng, and suma.

Precautions: Initial use may be marked by an increased heart rate. (Hachisu, Werbach)

Other Supplements and Substances

Glucosamine Sulfate

To begin a discussion of glucosamine (as well as chondroitin sulfate and MSM), we first have to look at the joints of the body and the cartilage within them. Our joints are structures which provide the various bones of our bodies attachment points and transitional junctions from one bony segment to another. Joints make movement possible by allowing motion between these bony segments. The joints of our bodies, depending on where they are located and what their purpose is, consist of a number of functional units: Cartilage, a joint capsule and cavity, synovium and synovial fluid, tendons, ligaments, etc. In regard to glucosamine, we need to look specifically at cartilage and its components. Cartilage, which is made up of collagen (fibers), proteoglycans, water and chondrocyte cells (which produce and maintain cartilage), is a major component of our joints. It works as a supportive mechanism within the joints, acting both as a cushion and shock absorber while allowing easy motion to occur over its smooth surfaces.

Glucosamine is a natural substance that is found throughout the human body, especially in the cartilage and connective tissues of our joints. Glucosamine is essentially a modified sugar molecule, made from glucose (a sugar) and from the amino acid glutamine. It is a critical component of cartilage health and resiliency. It is produced by the chondrocyte cells within the cartilage of our joints. It is a precursor to the production of GAGs (glycosaminoglycans – modified sugars), which are also manufactured by chondro-cytes and help retain water within the cartilage. It is a major component of hyaluronan (found in the proteo-glycan portion of cartilage), which helps provide a chemical linkage between sugars within cartilage and gives fluid within the joints lubricating ability. Unfortunately, glucosamine production decreases as we age, cartilage destruction and degeneration, typi-cally to a point where the joint is unable to keep pace or replace the cartilage being lost. This is why replace-ment of glucosamine in the body is so important!

There are essentially three forms of glu-cosamine: Glucosamine sulfate, glucosamine hydrochloride and NAG (N-acetylglucosamine). From a general replacement standpoint, glucosamine is what is needed and all three forms provide this. But there are important differences between these three. Most of the studies performed to date have looked more at glu-cosamine sulfate rather than the other two versions, although it appears that glucosamine hydrochloride is just as effective, possibly more so.

Glucosamine sulfate can be used for natural treatment of the various forms of arthritis, especially osteoarthritis. While glucosamine sulfate provides pain reduction and resolution, it is not considered specifically as a "first line" pain reliever. It appears that its pain relieving capabilities are from its effects as an anti-inflammatory. Reducing those chemical agents and enzymes which contribute to the inflammatory response.

While there are food sources that contain glu-cosamines within them, it is usually not bioavailable nor could they provide the necessary dosages which are required to achieve a therapeutic response. From this standpoint, the only viable alternative is the use of supplementation. In clinical and animal studies, the amount of supplementation needed to achieve a therapeutic response ranged from 1500 to 2000 mg per day in divided doses.

Precautions: Some glucosamine sulfates utilize salt (sodium chloride) as a stabilizer. If you are on a restricted salt diet for any reason, use the glucosamine hydrochloride form which does not contain salt.

Chondroitin Sulfate

Chondroitin sulfate is another major component of cartilage and other connective tissue. In cartilage it it part of proteoglycan and is integral to the production and makeup of the GAGs (glycosaminoglycans) that are so important to cartilage health. It is also present in the lining of blood vessels and the urinary bladder. Chondroitin sulfate is made up of repeating chains of sugar and like glucosamine sulfate, in the joints of the body it slows and stops the breakdown of cartilage and stimulates its repair. It decreases in the body as we age, and in the joints, decreases with cartilage degeneration and destruction.

The major source of chondroitin sulfate is from animal cartilage, such as cow (bovine), shark or whale cartilage. As with glucosamine, the only viable way of getting therapeutic dosages of chondroitin sulfate is through supplementation. In the United States, this can only be done with oral supplementation, while in Europe, injectable forms are also available.

There is a certain level of controversy surrounding the bioavailability and usage of chondroitin sulfate. Some of the clinical studies have presented opposing conclusions in regard to chondroitin sulfate's absorption and usage within the body and its uptake into the joints. Part of this controversy stems from the apparent molecule size of chondroitin sulfate, especially as compared with glucosamine. The other aspect of this controversy is from the brands and types of chondroitin sulfates used in the clinical studies themselves. These different brands had varying concentration levels and purity of chondroitin sulfate which in turn may have effected the clinical outcomes. Regardless of this controversy, it does appear that chondroitin sulfate is a valuable tool in certain conditions, especially arthritis and the pain associated with it. In my practice, I have arthritic patients who have used only glucosamine, others that have utilized only chondroitin sulfate, while another group has taken a combinations of these two substances. I have found that all of these patients achieved decreased pain levels and improved joint mobility, however, the group taking the combination of chondroitin sulfate with glucosamine achieved the best results.

Conditions which may be helped with chondroitin sulfate include arthritis (especially osteoarthritis), atherosclerosis, high cholesterol and kidney stones.

Precautions: Nausea may occur at very high doses (more than10 grams per day).

MSM

MSM stands for "methyl-sulfonyl-methane" and is from the sulfur family. It is an organic form of sulfur and a metabolite of DMSO (dimethy-sulfoxide - *DMSO will be discussed in the section on topical pain relievers). MSM occurs widely in nature, being found in both plants and animals, and plays an essential role in human nutrition. Sulfur is a trace element stored within every cell of our bodies. Its highest concentrations are found in our muscles, bones, joints, skin, hair and nails. It is necessary for the production of collagen, the primary constituent of cartilage and connective in the body. In connective tissue, it provides the disulfide bonds between the proteins which hold the connective tissue together.

The major sources of sulfur, and thus MSM, are from the foods which contain sulfur. Included in this large group are many fruits and vegetables. Examples are: Brussels sprouts, corn, garlic, legumes, onions, peppers and tomatoes. Other sources of MSM include soybeans, fish, meats, eggs, whole grains and wheat germ.

MSM is also found in a group of sulfur amino acids that include methionine, cysteine, cystine, taurine and glutathione. There are also other substances which contain sulfur. Examples of some of these include: Vitamin B1, biotin, alpha lipoic acid, coenzyme A, insulin, glucosamine and chondroitin. As you can see, we can obtain MSM from many foods, it is however, lost in the processing of foods.

Conditions which may be helped with MSM include allergies, arthritis (osteoarthritis, rheumatoid arthritis, systemic lupus erythematosus, etc.), asthma, cancer, colitis, constipation, diabetes, heartburn, inflammation, muscle soreness, muscle cramps, pain, parasites, skin and hair conditions.

Precautions: Essentially none.

Essential Fatty Acids

Our society, especially here in the United States, has an ongoing war going against fat. There is a general assumption that all fats are bad for us, however, this is incorrect. The fact is, there are "good fats" and "bad fats." The "good fats" are called Essential Fatty Acids (EFAs) and are critical to our health. EFAs are the fatty acids which cannot be produced by our bodies and must be taken in through our diets. EFAs are basic building blocks in our bodies and makes up fats and oils. Essential fatty acids are found in high concentrations in the brain and throughout the body. Every cell needs EFAs. They are critical for the repair and rebuilding of cells as well as the production of new cells.

Our bodies use EFAs to produce prostaglandins (hormone-like substances that act as chemical messengers and regulate various body processes). Essential fatty acids are very important to the health of our joints, providing basic nutrients and fulfilling vital roles for the cartilage and synovial fluid. EFAs are very valuable, both directly and indirectly, in controlling pain, inflammation and swelling.

There are two categories of essential fatty acids: the Omega-3 and Omega-6 fatty acids. Of these two, Omega-6 fatty acids include linoleic and gamma linoleic acids. Omega-3 fatty acids include alpha-linolenic (LNA), eicosapentaenoic acid (EPA) and docosahexaenoic acid (DHA).

Sources of these essential fatty acids can be found in many types of oils. For the Omega-6 group, sources include raw nuts and seeds, legumes and unsaturated vegetable oils (such as borage oil, grape seed oil, primrose oil, sesame oil and soybean oil). For the Omega-3 fatty acids, sources include cold water fish (such as salmon and tuna), fish oil and other vegetable oils (such as canola, flaxseed and walnut).

Even though we can get the needed essential fatty acids from our diets, the best way to get specific therapeutic doses of these critical fatty acids is through supplementation. This becomes very important when you are addressing disease processes and for general health and prevention since you can control the amounts you get day-to-day. A number of companies produce both singular and combinations of these essential fatty acids for your use.

EFA's have positive effects on a great many disorders and conditions. This is especially true for cardiovascular diseases and related disorders. There are many conditions in which essential fatty acids can prove beneficial for and effective in treating. These include: Acne, alcohol-related disorders, anti-aging, arthritis (osteoarthritis, rheumatoid arthritis, etc.), asthma, atherosclerosis, attention deficit disorder, cancer, candida, cardiovascular disease and related-disorders, cholesterol reduction, cystic fibrosis, diabetes, eczema, hair loss, high blood pressure, hypertension, infertility, menstrual cramps, multiple sclerosis, pregnancy, premenstrual syndrome, prenatal development, psoriasis, reduce risk of blood clot formation, skin disorders, triglyceride reduction, weight loss and weight changes. Essential fatty acids are critical to prevention of many diseases and for maintaining general health.

Precautions: Essentially none. You may want to increase your intake of Vitamin E to help prevent peroxidation of these sensitive fatty acids in the body. Many supplements already contain added E so be sure to check your supplement labels.

Water

Water is an underrated resource, one that we take for granted on a daily basis. Our bodies are made up mostly of water (approximately 2/3) and yet many of us do not replenish this critical fluid each day. Why does this happen when water is abundantly available and accessible? Sadly, too many of us have replaced drinking water with other fluids such as coffee, tea, and soda pop.

Water is critical to our very survival. Drinking eight, eight ounce glasses of water each day is necessary to ensure that we maintain optimum health. Water is necessary to perform so many functions within the human body that naming them all is impossible. Some examples of the actions of water is its necessity for most chemical reactions, the transportation of nutrients and waste products, for digestion and absorption of nutrients, for maintaining our body temperature, for proper circulatory function, etc.

Water is critical to the proper functioning of the body. We must keep hydrated. Dehydration need not be a full blown clinical state. Even low levels of fluid decrease can lead to clinical problems. Dehydration can cause dysfunction in the systems of the body. An example is in the musculoskeletal system - the bones, muscle and joints of our bodies. Without adequate water to our muscles and joints, we create an environment in which they cannot function properly. This can lead to pain within those involved muscles and joints. In my practice, I have found that immediate hydration over the first 24 hours can prove invaluable in reducing pain levels in many conditions, especially those involving arthritis, sprains, strains, tendonitis, bruises, etc.

Enzymes

SOD (Superoxide Dismutase)

Superoxide Dismutase is an important enzyme whose usefulness is derived from its antioxidant capability; specifically with the neutralization of the free radical superoxide (superoxide is one of the most damaging free radicals found in nature). SOD, because of its capability, is vital for cellular health, especially as it pertains to protecting and reducing the rate of cell destruction. As with many protective compounds within our bodies, it decrease as we age. This translates to loss of its protective strength as the blood levels decrease.

There are two varieties of SOD available. They are a Copper/Zinc SOD and a Manganese SOD. These two substances act upon cells in two different ways. Copper/zinc SOD works on and protects the cytoplasm of the cell. This is important because much of the free radicals (damaging agents) is produced in the cytoplasm by metabolic activity. Manganese SOD works within the cell to protect the mitochondria (a mitochondria is a cells energy producing mechanism and also contains genetic information).

Sources of SOD include broccoli, barley grass, Brussels sprouts, cabbage, and wheat grass. It is also found in the majority of green plants.

SOD can be used in anti-aging applications, arthritis (osteo and rheumatoid arthritis), cancer and as an overall anti-oxidant.

Precautions: Make sure that the SOD you are taking is enteric coated. This coating protects the tablet from being broken down in the stomach, so it is broken down and absorbed in the small intestine.

Digestive/Food/Metabolic Enzymes

There are three different categories of enzymes in this section: Digestive, food and metabolic enzymes. While these enzymes are derived from a variety of sources and perform many different functions; they also share many similar actions and functions at the same time. This is especially true in regard to their pain relieving capability. It is important to remember that these enzymes will come from both external sources (food) and internal sources (body chemicals, body structures and organs). The majority of these enzymes are also available in supplement form, which may be absolutely necessary for you to bring their levels up within the body. We will begin with some basic definitions and classifications.

Important note: You will find a basic overlap of the enzymes types named in the following classifications, even though they will be found under different categories. This is due to their origins, from external food sources versus coming from inside the body. Don't let this confuse you. Our interest is in how these enzymes can work within our bodies to provide either direct and/or indirect pain relief.

Digestive enzymes: This group is also known as the "Pancreatic Enzymes." These enzymes are those that are secreted within our bodies, from the mouth, stomach, small intestine and pancreas. The enzymes of this group include the following: Amylase, chymotrypsin, lipase, pancreatin, protease and trypsin. There are approximately 22 enzymes within this group, some which are very prominent and others that play lesser roles. We will focus on the main ones listed above.

Food enzymes: This group are also known as the "Plant Enzymes." These enzymes are present in all raw foods and are critical for proper digestion of our food. As you can tell from the name, these enzymes actually enter our body as part of the food sources that we are consuming. Examples of these enzymes would be papain and bromelain from pineapple. They can also be taken as supplements, as mentioned earlier.

Metabolic enzymes: This group of enzymes is enormous with literally hundreds of thousands of them found within the body. These enzymes are critical to the functions and actions of the millions of biochemical reactions taking place in our bodies every day. Examples of the functions that these enzymes perform include helping the blood to coagulate, eliminating carbon dioxide from the lungs (from respiratory enzymes), assisting the removal of waste from the kidneys and liver, etc. Examples of these enzymes include SOD and catalase.

Enzymes are vital to our lives, without them we would perish very rapidly. They are active all the time, performing a multitude of chemical functions and activities that are necessary for normal performance. Enzymes work at every level in our bodies, from the cellular level (in individual cells) through the various systems (gastrointestinal system). We take in enzymes each time we eat. Our whole foods contain many different enzymes. These plant enzymes initiate digestion of our food stuff, proteins, carbohydrates and fat digestion. Internally, our bodies produce enzymes to finish these breakdown processes and fuel millions of biochemical reactions.

The following is a brief description of the enzymes that have been previously listed. Remember, these are only a small group of the many enzymes working within us.

1. Amylase: Found in the saliva, pancreatic and intestinal juices. It breaks down carbohydrates. Different types of amylase (such as lactase, maltase and sucrase) break down different sugar types.

2. Bromelain: Found in the pineapple and papaya fruits, it aids in the breakdown and digestion of protein.

3. Cellulase: Found in many raw foods, it is used for the digestion of soluble fiber into smaller units.

4. Chymotrypsin: This is a digestive enzyme is found in the intestinal juices. It helps to break down and digest proteins.

5. Lipase: Found in the stomach and pancreatic juices helps digest fat. It is also found within fats in foods.

6. Papain: Found in the pineapple and papaya fruits, it aids in the breakdown and digestion of protein.

7. Pepsin: Is a proteolytic enzyme found within the stomach. It aids in the digestion and breakdown of protein.

8. Protease: Found in the stomach, pancreatic and intestinal juices. It helps break down and digest protein. Included in this group is the proteolytic enzyme pepsin.

9. Trypsin: Is found in the intestinal juices. It helps break down and digest proteins.

Enzymes can found in many different foods, from both plant and animal sources. In the plant group, raw sources are best and include the majority of fruits and some vegetables.

Conditions in which enzymes can prove valuable to prevent, reverse and treat include the following: Acne, allergies, arthritis, asthma, healing broken bones, bruises, cancer, candidiasis, cardiovascular disease, diabetes, fibroids, gallbladder disorders, gastric disorders (gastritis, ulcers, etc.), headaches, herpes, hyperactivity syndromes (ADD), insomnia, intervertebral disc disorders, intestinal disorders, kidney stones, menopausal symptoms, mental disorders, osteoporosis, parasites, premenstrual syndrome, seizures, skin disorders, sprains and strains, tendonitis and weight problems. This is not an all inclusive list either. Enzymes can, and do impact most all conditions and diseases to some degree or another.

Precautions: Whether changing our whole food eating patterns to increase the enzymes we get each day or through supplementation, it is important to know what type of enzymes you need and the dosages. This is especially important when you have a diagnosed disease or condition. In regard to pain control, it is very important to utilize the services of a health care professional who understands and utilizes enzyme therapy in the treatment of pain and its related conditions.

Amino Acids

Amino acids are the building blocks of proteins and are critical to life. There are 22 amino acids of which eight are considered essential. Essential amino acids are those that cannot be produced in the body and therefore must be supplied daily through the diet. For the body to utilize the various amino acids, they must all be present and in the correct amounts. If any amino acid is not present in the sufficient amounts, it can in turn effect the other amino acids uptake and usage. For our purposes, we will specifically be addressing just two amino acids out of this group in this section. They are: DL-phenylalanine and tryptophan (in its available over-the-counter form called 5-hydroxy-tryptophan). This is because of the evidence available in regard to their pain relieving capabilities. It is important to remember that the other amino acids, especially the essential forms, are all important for general health and in addressing diseases and conditions within the body. All of these amino acids may impact pain within the body, in both indirect and direct ways.

DL-Phenylalanine

DL-phenylalanine, also known as DLPA, is a form of one of the eight essential amino acids, phenylalanine. DLPA is made up of the basic amino acid phenylalanine and combinations of equal parts of two forms within its makeup; the synthetic form (designated the D-form) and the natural form (designated the L-form). It is from the combination of these two forms that it gets the designation of "DL." There is also an "L" form available commercially. Both the "D-form" and the "DL-form" have the capability of to act as pain relievers.

DL-phenylalanine acts on the central nervous system within the body. It can decrease pain, aid in memory and learning and can suppress the appetite. In regard to pain, DLPA works in producing and activating endorphins within the body. Through this, it can assist the body in reducing pain. DLPA can be very useful for chronic pain and can become more effective over time.

Conditions that DLPA can help with include chronic pain, especially with neck pain, low back pain, back pain, osteoarthritis, rheumatoid arthritis, migraine headaches, postoperative pain, leg and muscle cramps and neuralgia. Other conditions that it can be effective for include depression, menstrual cramps, obesity, Parkinson's disease and schizophrenia.

Precautions: Phenylalanine and DLPA should not be taken by pregnant women and people who have PKU (phenylketonuria – an inborn error of metabolism in which phenylalanine is not converted in the body into tyrosine with devastating results). Phenylalanine may cause a rise in blood pressure and should not be taken by those with cardiovascular disease, high blood pressure or hypertension without first consulting a doctor.

Tryptophan/5-Hydroxy-Tryptophan

Tryptophan is one of the essential amino acids and is a critical precursor for the neurotransmitter serotonin (serotonin is necessary for normal sleep, the transfer of nerve signals from cell to cell and for our mental health status). Tryptophan is necessary for the production of Vitamin B1 (thiamine). Tryptophan can reduce pain sensitivity, provide mood stability, reduce anxiety and tension, reduce depression and can help with appetite control. It may also help with migraine headaches, hypertension, vascular disorders, addiction disorders (such as alcoholism) and nausea.

In 1989, because of problems relating to a bad batch of tryptophan, the FDA caused all tryptophan supplements to be removed from store shelves. In the last year or so, another form of tryptophan has become available. It is called **5-hydroxy-tryptophan (5-HTP)** and is the first stage of tryptophan's biochemical breakdown in the body. It is derived from the African botanical *Griffonia simplicifolia* and therefore is available as an over-the-counter supplement which great news for the general public! We again have access to supplemental tryptophan.

Natural sources of tryptophan include bananas, brown rice, cottage cheese, fish, milk, meats, peanuts and soybeans. For specific usages, as in the treatment of particular conditions or as a sleep aid, use the 5-hydroxy-tryptophan supplement form in dosages ranging from 50 to 150 mg twice daily.

Precaution: It is not advisable to supplement 5-HTP in dosages more than one gram (1,000 mg) per day. Because of the conversion to serotonin, supplementation of 5-HTP can cause drowsiness especially at higher dosages.

Herbals

There are many herbal substances which can impact pain. Some of these will impact the pain directly, while others work in an indirect fashion (i.e. on inflammation, muscle spasms, sprain and strains, bruises, etc). Herbs have been used medicinally for centuries to treat a large variety of maladies. Until the advent of "modern medicine," herbal therapies were the mainstay treatment for disease in many cultures. The scientific knowledge base for herbals is incredibly extensive and there are a number of excellent texts that deal with this subject in depth. Information has been gathered over literally centuries. In recent years, herbs have been the subject of many clinical trials. Herbs have amazing properties and capabilities, many of them medicinal and pharmacological in nature. Because of these incredible capabilities, herbs are an area that I highly recommend for study. There are many types and varieties of herbs available commercially and they come from around the globe.

For this section, I have included a mixture of the different herbs that are available. However, due to constraints of space, I have listed only 20 different herbs. Please remember that we are only skimming the surface here and that there are literally hundreds of herbs which have medicinal value for a number of medical conditions. In this regard, the capability of herbal therapies to resolve and impact these diseases and conditions can, in turn, decrease and resolve pain. Some herbs that are discussed in this section will crossover into the homeopathic section. These will be noted with each herb that this is true.

Arnica

Arnica is a well known perennial plant that has been used medicinally for hundreds of years in internal as well as external (topical) preparations. There are various species that have been used medicinally with perhaps the most well known being *Arnica montana* (scientific name). Arnica has been used in both herbal and homeopathic preparations for its analgesic and anti-inflammatory effects.

Conditions that Arnica can be used for include: Arthritis, bronchitis and cough, the common cold, inflammatory conditions (skin, mouth, pharynx, joints, muscles, etc.), as a mild analgesic, blunt injuries, etc.

Precautions: Arnica has the potential for negative qualities which have led some authorities to recommend that it not be taken internally. From a toxicology standpoint, Arnica is considered poisonous. This occurs only with overdoses which can irritate mucous membranes, and cause stomach pain, diarrhea and vomiting. At very high doses, Arnica can cause gastroenteritis, dyspnea and cardiac arrest/palsy. These problems usually only happen when Arnica is wild crafted (picked directly from nature), formulated and/or used by those that do not understand its dangers and usage.

In most commercial preparations, the dosages are typically low and are safe to consume orally, especially with the homeopathic preparations. For safety reasons with taking Arnica orally, it is always advisable to seek the advice of a health care professional. This is especially true if you have a diagnosed conditions, and a history of cardiovascular disease, hypertension or other heart-related problems.

Black Cohosh

Black Cohosh, scientific name, *Cimicifuga racemosa*, has purported estrogenic effects through the binding of estrogen receptor sites and its effects on other female hormones. It has been used traditionally in the treatment of dysmenorrhea, dyspepsia, rheumatisms, premenstrual syndrome and menopausal climacteric complaints (hot flashes, night sweats, mood changes, etc).

Other conditions in which Black Cohosh may also prove valuable include: Asthma, coughs, high blood pressure and snake bites. It is part of the nervine group of herbals and has proven anti-spasmodic effects to smooth muscle. In this regard, it can prove to have indirect pain relieving effects.

Precautions: This herb should not be taken during pregnancy as it may induce miscarriage and premature birth. Overdose may cause nausea, vomiting, dizziness, headache, nervous system and visual disturbances and increased perspiration. However, no health hazards or side effects are known when properly administered or used in designated therapeutic dosages.

Blue Vervain

Blue Vervain contains a number of chemical agents, one of which is verbenalin (a glucoside). Verbenalin has moderate parasympathetic properties and works on the sensory nerves leading to the brain, providing a tranquilizing sensation to the mind, where there is restlessness and agitation. Because of this, it can be useful as a sleep aid for those suffering from insomnia and is known as the "natural tranquilizer." Blue Vervain stimulates nerve endings, blood vessels and the salivary glands. It can reduce fevers and colds. It can also be used as an expectorant and is helpful with coughs, pneumonia and asthma.

Blue Vervain has definite analgesic and anti-inflammatory activity. In this capacity, it has been used for hundreds of years as part of folk medicine. It has a general calming effect on the nervous system and by normalizing this system, can reduce pain.

Blue Vervain can be helpful for arthritic conditions, asthma, anxiety, bronchitis, colds, convulsions, coughs, digestive conditions, fevers, flu, headaches, hyperactivity, indigestion, insomnia, lung congestion, muscle and spinal pain, nervousness and nervous conditions (restlessness, etc), pain, pneumonia, seizures, and sore throat.

Precautions: As with all herbs, caution must be taken not take too much within 24 hours.

Boswellia

Boswellia is a tree that is found in dry, hilly areas of India. Its common name is *Salai guggal*. Boswellia has been historically used in Ayurvedic medicine in India. It has been recommended for a variety of conditions including arthritis, diarrhea, dysentery, pulmonary disease and ringworm.

Studies have shown that boswellic acids, one of the active components of Boswellia, have an anti-inflammatory action. Boswellia inhibits pro-inflammatory mediators in the body. For this reason, it is used in many conditions in which there is an inflammatory component. Boswellia tends to be well tolerated by the stomach, unlike traditional NSAIDs.

Conditions that Boswellia may prove valuable in are osteoarthritis, rheumatoid arthritis and bursitis.

Precautions: Boswellia is generally safe. In very high doses and overdoses, it may cause diarrhea, nausea or a skin rash.

Burdock

Burdock, known scientifically as *Arctium lappa*, is widely found in Europe and Asia and has a long history of usage in these areas. Burdock has been used for a wide range of activities, including antipyretic (fever reducing), antimicrobial, antitumor, and as a diuretic and diaphorectic (promoting perspiration). It has historically been used as a blood purifier to clear the bloodstream of toxins.

There are a variety of conditions that Burdock has uses for including: Fever, infection, cancer, fluid retention and kidney stones. Other ailments include colds, gout, rheumatism, stomach ailments, psoriasis and as a laxative. In chinese medicine, burdock is used with a combination with other herbs to treat colds, sore throats and tonsillitis. Burdock is also useful for cankers, boils, abscesses, etc.

Precautions: Burdock has a small potential to cause an allergic skin reaction in those sensitive to Burdock. In rare occasions, Burdock root tea poisoning has been documented.

Cayenne

Cayenne has been used medicinally for centuries. The Cayenne plant is very closely related to bell peppers, jalapenos and other peppers. This "hot" fruit is helpful for a variety of conditions. Cayenne contains a number of chemical compounds. One group are the capsaicinoids, of which capsaicin is one of its chief components. It is well known as a circulatory tonic (improve circulation).

Cayenne can be used both internally and externally as a topical agent. Internally, Cayenne is used for gastrointestinal disorders (stomach aches, stomach cramping and pains, gas, etc.), loss of appetite, dyspepsia, diarrhea, alcoholism, malaria fever, yellow fever and other fevers. It can be used as a preventive and prophylactically for a number of cardiovascular conditions including arteriosclerosis, stroke and heart disease. Cayenne's topical aspects will be discussed under the section on Topical Approaches.

Precautions: Very high doses of Cayenne taken internally, especially at the higher heat units (100,000 plus) and over an extended period of time, may cause ulcers or gastritis.

Chamomile

Chamomile is one of the best known cure-alls and has been used medicinally for many years. It is a bitter tonic with many proven properties. These include its actions as an antispasmodic (muscle relaxation), anti-inflammatory and for its sedative effects. The other proven actions of Chamomile include its effects on gastrointestinal complaints, antibacterial, and antimycotic (anti-fungal) effects. The traditional role of Chamomile is as a bitter, including its stimulating effect on the liver. Chamomile has shown to have antitumor effects and this aspect is being researched for cancer treatment. It also promotes wound healing.

Conditions in which Chamomile can be useful

include bronchitis, canker sores, common colds, coughs, diarrhea, eczema, gingivitis, inflammatory conditions, insomnia, irritable bowel syndrome, insomnia, liver and gall bladder conditions, loss of appetite, peptic ulcer, wound and burn healing, etc.

Chamomile has anti-inflammatory and antispasmodic effects, especially in the gastrointestinal system. In this regard, it can have pain relieving effects in an indirect fashion.

Precautions: Rare allergic reactions have been reported. Persons with allergies to ragweed, aster and chrysanthemum should avoid use of Chamomile.

Devil's Claw

The medicinal parts of Devil's Claw are derived from the dried tubers and roots from this plant that grows in Namibia and South Africa. Devil's Claw has been used as a folk remedy by Africans for a variety of diseases, especially for rheumatism. The major chemical component of Devil's Claw is harpagoside which is believed to be responsible for its anti-inflammatory effects. Devil's Claw acts as an appetite stimulant and has choleretic (stimulating bile production), and analgesic effects. It may also reduce blood pressure and decrease heart rate.

Conditions in which Devil's Claw can prove beneficial include arteriosclerosis, arthritis, heartburn, indigestion, joint pain, rheumatoid arthritis, liver and gallbladder complaints, and loss of appetite.

Precautions: Caution should be taken if stomach or duodenal ulcers are present. Devil's Claw may irritate or aggravate these conditions by its promotion of stomach acid.

English Horsemint

This plant is common in all of Europe and the medicinal part if the dried herb. English Horsemint has carminative (reduces gas and bowel pains) and stimulant effects. In Europe, English Horsemint has been used for all kinds of pain, especially headaches.

English Horsemint has been used for digestive disorders and arthritic pains. No known precautions are known in regard to the proper usage and with therapeutic dosages.

Feverfew

Feverfew is known botanically as *Tanacetum parthenium* and is a member of the daisy family. It is found all over Europe. Feverfew has a long history, even being mentioned in Greek literature as a remedy for inflammation and menstrual discomfort. The active compounds in Feverfew are known as sequiterpene lactones. Of this group, the most important is parthenolide, which is critical for therapeutic interventions. It may impede or slow down platelet aggregation, prostaglandin synthesis and the release histamines.

Conditions in which Feverfew can prove effective are aches and pains, allergies, arthritis, fever, migraine headaches and rheumatic disease.

Precautions: Feverfew is not recommended during pregnancy. It may cause mild gastrointestinal upset.

Horse Chestnut

Chestnuts have been used in folk and traditional medicines for centuries. Horse Chestnut has been used as a traditional remedy for arthritis and rheumatism. Horse Chestnut has been found to decrease venous capillary permeability and tonifies the circulatory system. It can improve edema and chronic deep vein incompetence. The bark of the Horse Chestnut has been found to possess anti-inflammatory activity.

Conditions in which Horse Chestnut can prove effective are eczema, superficial and deep varicose veins, leg pains, painful injuries, sprains, bruising and pain syndromes of the spine, phlebitis and thrombophlebitis, hemorrhoids, spastic pains before and during menstruation. It has also been used for arthritis and rheumatism.

Precautions: Horse Chestnut has the potential to be toxic and has the capability to be a very dangerous herb, thus it must be used with caution. In fact, the FDA has declared Horse Chestnut to be unsafe. Depending on which source you study, horse chestnut should not be taken internally or it can be taken safely in specific therapeutic doses. Usually Horse Chestnut is included in a "vein tea" formula along with other herbs and is in a small dose.

Kava Kava

Kava Kava has been receiving a lot of media attention over the last year or so. Kava has a number of interesting properties that have been clinically proven. Its scientific name is *Piper methysticum* and it comes from the South Pacific. There are many varieties of the Kava plant with both black and white grades available. There are a number of chemical compounds which contribute to Kava's medicinal effects. These are called Kavalactones or pyrones. Kava has a demonstrated anti-anxiety effect. It also has an analgesic effect thought to come from "non-opiate pathways."

Conditions in which Kava can help include anxiety states, insomnia, menopausaul symptoms, nervousness, obsessive-compulsive disorders, pain syndromes (headaches, neck pain, back pain, toothache and others), panic disorders, premenstrual tension, stress relief and temporomandibular syndrome.

Precautions: Excessive usage can lead to a skin disorder characterized by a scaly rash and eye irritation. Do not take if you have Parkinson's Disease, are severely depressed, pregnant or nursing. Caution needs to be taken if you are concurrently taking other medications that have similar effects. As with all calming/sedating herbals, use caution if you will be operating heavy machinery.

Licorice

Licorice, scientific name, *Glycyrrhiza glabra,* has been used medicinally for literally centuries, especially in the Chinese culture. It is grown in many areas of Europe and Asia. Licorice is produced from the harvested roots of the plant. As with most plants, licorice contains a number of valuable chemical compounds. One of its prominent chemicals is the glycoside glycyrrhizin. Licorice is an expectorant, anti-ulcerogenic (ulcer reducing), antibacterial, antiviral, anti-arrhythmic (normalizing heart rhythms), anti-inflammatory and as an anti-arthritic. It may also have anti-spasmodic effects to muscle. In cases with elevated or high blood pressure, that are not diagnosed as hypertensive, the DGL (deglycyrrhizinated) form of Licorice may be taken with a doctor's monitoring.

Conditions in which Licorice can help treat include arthritis, asthma, bronchitis, canker sores, chronic fatigue syndrome, cough, eczema, fibromyalgia, gastritis, heartburn, indigestion, herpes simplex, peptic ulcer disease. It may also have value in the treatment of SLE (Lupus).

Precautions: Licorice should not be taken during pregnancy. Excessive licorice intake can cause hypernatremia (sodium increase and retention), edema (fluid retention), and an increase in blood pressure leading to hypertension. Patients with preexisting renal disease (kidney), hepatic disease (liver – especially with chronic hepatitis, cirrhosis and cholestatic diseases of the liver) or cardiovascular disease are contraindicated from taking licorice.

Peony

Known scientifically as *Paeonia officinalis*, Peony is a perennial plant which grows wild in South Europe and is cultivated in other areas around the world including Portugal, Hungary and Asia Minor. It is used as an antispasmodic, diuretic and a sedative. In folk medicine Peony root has been used for neuralgia, migraines, epilepsy and whooping cough.

Conditions in which Peony can be used include ailments of the respiratory tract, asthma, fissures, gout, eclampsia and rheumatoid arthritis.

Precautions: When used with proper administration of therapeutic dosages, Peony can be safe and effective. However, the Peony plant can be poisonous and should not be used without medical supervision. Over dosage can cause vomiting, colic and diarrhea.

Rosemary

Rosemary is a perennial shrub which is cultivated worldwide. Its scientific name is *Rosmarinus officinalis*. It is used widely as a culinary spice. Medicinally and in folk medicine, rosemary leaves have been used effectively in Europe and China to treat headaches and stomach pains. The major chemical component is a volatile oil from the leaves. It has been found that this oil contributes the calming and soothing effects to tense muscles and nerves. It has been shown that Rosemary is an antispasmodic, mild analgesic, carminative, diuretic, digestive remedy and nervine. Rosemary is also a powerful antioxidant which indirectly can hasten healing in the body and help prevent free radical damage resulting from inflammation or other effects from injury.

Conditions in which rosemary may be of value in treating include circulatory problems, high blood pressure, liver and gallbladder problems, loss of appetite and Rheumatism. Topically is can increase blood flow to an area and act as an analgesic.

Precautions: Over dosage of Rosemary's volatile oil can cause vomiting, spasms, kidney irritation. Caution should be taken if pregnant.

Skullcap

Skullcap has been used as an antispasmodic, anti-epileptic, antibacterial, diuretic and can promote the flow of bile. It is one of the best herbs to treat nervous disorders from insomnia to hysteria. It is an excellent nervine, is very calming and soothing to the nerves and has been used as a sedative. Skullcap has an interesting history in regard to pain relief. In some cultures, it is strongly recommended for the relief of headaches and related pains.

Conditions in which Skullcap can be used include alcoholism, convulsions, coughs, epilepsy, headaches, hysteria, indigestion, insomnia, nervous diseases, nervous tension, neuralgia, pain, restlessness, rheumatism and stress.

Precautions: When used with proper administration of therapeutic dosages, Skullcap can be safe and effective. Overdoses may cause vomiting and diarrhea.

Turmeric

Turmeric, known by the scientific name *Curcuma domestica*, is a perennial which comes from India and is also cultivated in southern Asia. The roots and rhizome of the plant are used medicinally. Turmeric has a long history of usage in Indian Ayurvedic medicine. In Ayurvedic and folk medicine, Turmeric has been used for a variety of disorders including dyspeptic disorders, diarrhea, fever, dropsy, bronchitis, colds, worms, kidney inflammation and cystitis. Other uses have included headaches, flatulence, upper abdominal pains, colic and amenorrhea. It can also be used externally for bruising, eye infections, inflammation of the oral mucosa, inflammatory skin conditions and infected wounds. Turmeric also provides antioxidant protective benefits.

Conditions in which Turmeric is used include atherosclerosis, bursitis, inflammation, liver and gallbladder complaints, loss of appetite, rheumatoid arthritis. Other uses include amenorrhea, colic, flatulence, headaches and upper abdominal pains. It can also be used externally for bruising, eye infections, inflammation of the oral mucosa, inflammatory skin conditions and infected wounds.

Precautions: Stomach complaints may occur with extended use or with over dosage.

Valerian

Valerian, scientific name *Valeriana officinalis*, is a widely distributed perennial found in North America, Europe and Asia. There are three distinct chemical compounds associated with Valerian: A volatile oil, a small number of alkaloids and a group of esters called valepotriates (which are considered the most important chemical group in valerian). Valerian is another herb which has long been used historically for a host of medical problems including digestive disorders, liver problems, nausea and nervous conditions. It has definite sedative effects and is an anti-spasmodic (muscle relaxant).

Conditions in which valerian can be used include colic, epilepsy, fainting, headaches, hysteria, insomnia, lack of concentration, menopause, mental strain, muscle cramps, neuralgia, nervous cardiopathy, nervousness, nervous stomach, neurasthenia, premenstrual tension, restlessness, sleeping disorders, stress, uterine spasticity, and tonicity.

Precautions: Valerian is generally safe, but caution should be used if other central nervous system depressants are concurrently used.

White Willow Bark

White willow bark comes from the white willow tree. The bark is used medicinally and contains its active chemical constituents. White willow bark is the original source of salicin, the forerunner of aspirin, though weaker in activity. It has been used down through the ages a combat pain of many different types, including rheumatism, headaches, fever, arthritis, gout and angina. The usage of White Willow is mentioned in ancient Greek and Egyptian texts. It has analgesic properties, antipyretic, disinfectant and antiseptic properties.

Conditions that White Willow Bark include arthritis (especially osteoarthritis and rheumatoid arthritis), bursitis, fever, headaches and pain syndromes throughout the body.

Precautions: Stomach complaints can occur large and/or extended doses. Caution needs to be taken if ulcer disease is present.

Wood Betony

Wood betony, scientific name is *Betonica officinalis*, has been used for over 400 hundred years for a large variety of maladies. Its acts as an astringent, bitter tonic, disinfectant, expectorant, nervine, sedative and tranquilizer. It may have hypotensive actions. In folk medicine is has ben used as an anti-diarrheal and a carmative.

Conditions that wood betony can prove useful include aches and pains, anxiety, asthma, bronchitis, coughs headaches, nervousness and neuralgia.

Precautions: Avoid during pregnancy as this herb may act as a uterine stimulant.

Homeopathics

Homeopathy has been in use for over 200 years and is used worldwide. In Europe and Britain, it has been integrated as a mainstream therapeutic approach, while in the United States it is regaining popularity and usage. Homeopathy is a therapeutic method which is based on the "Law of Similars." The Law of Similars is the fundamental principle of homeopathy and basically states that a parallel action or similarity of action can be achieved between the toxic potential of a substance and its therapeutic action. In layman's terms, this means that "like cures like." Essentially, by taking a particular homeopathic substance in a tiny dose, a substance that can cause or create the same symptoms that the person is experiencing, you will in fact relieve the patient's symptoms and resolve the condition. Please note that I am stating this simplistically, and that defining all the aspects of Homeopathy can easily encompass a book. It achieves its response by using medically active substances at weak or infinitesimal doses.

Homeopathic doses are made by successive steps of diluting or attenuating a base substance into a weaker and weaker dose to achieve specific potency levels. The dilutions are called "Homeopathic Potencies." There are two levels of dilution. One level is the centesimal scale in which are one part of a substance is diluted with a hundred parts of distilled water or ethyl alcohol. This process is repeated again and again to achieve the specific dosage. The centesimal scale is most common in the United States is represented by the letter "c." The other level is the decimal scale in which dilutions are sequentially diluted at one part to ten part ratio. This scale using the letter "x" to identify it. The greater the dilution, the greater the potency, thus a 6c is less potent that a 30c. Homeopathy remedies are very individualized, with the treatment protocols based on the individual's symptoms and needs. As with the herbal section, there are some homeopathic remedies that use plant and/or herbs, however, the therapeutic approach and dosages are very different. As with herbal medicine, Homeopathy is an excellent natural-based approach to complaints and disease.

In this section, we will be listing homeopathic substances that can relieve pain. The different substances have been drawn from a variety of sources and then verified through the "Homeopathic Materia Medica." I have listed ten substances here. As with the herbal section, there are numerous other homeopathic substances and remedies which can cause direct and indirect pain relief. For more information on Homeopathy, please see the Recommended Reading List at the back of this book.

Agar

Agar, also known as Aga, goes by the scientific names *Agaricus muscarius* and *Amanita muscaria*. This substance is a fungi (mushroom/toadstool) that grows in Europe, Asia and United States. Agar has been used by medicine men in the past as a hallucinogen and in ritualistic ceremonies. It has been used in folk medicine for headaches and nervous twitching. This fungi is highly toxic (See Precautions), and should only be harvested by knowlegable professionals.

Conditions in which agar have proved helpful are anxiety, alcohol poisoning, fever, headaches, joint pains and neuralgia. It also has hallucinogenic qualities.

Precautions: As with many mushrooms, this drug is highly toxic. Signs of poisoning can include dizziness, vomiting, abdominal pain and muscle cramps. Severe overdoses can lead to confusions, coordination problems, maniac attacks, unconsciousness, coma and death. Please realize we are discussing a huge intake of this substance to create the overdose levels (from 10 grams to over a 100 grams). In homeopathic dosages and preparations, this substance is therapeutically safe.

Belladonna

Belladonna, also known as the "Deadly Nightshade," is scientifically known as *Atropa belladonna.* This is another plant whose poisonous properties are well known and yet has been well utilized in both herbal and homeopathic medicine. It has an interesting background in folklore, especially in regard to its use in witchcraft, magic and as a hallucinogen in ritualistic ceremonies. The poisoning aspects of belladonna are very similar to the symptoms of scarlet fever and it is from this that homeopathy created a remedy. As with Agar, belladonna is highly toxic, and should only be harvested by knowlegable professionals.

Conditions in which belladonna can be used for a variety of complaints including arrhythmia, cardiac insufficiency, ear ache, fever, gastrointestinal and bile duct pain, headaches, liver and gallbladder complaints, menstrual pain, muscle pain, muscle cramps and spasms, nervous heart complaints, organ muscle relaxation, teething pain and vascular congestion.

Precautions: This is a poisonous substance and

precautions need to be taken with its usage. In properly administered homeopathic dosages, for the appropriate complaints, belladonna is safe. Overdoses can lease to hallucinations, delirium, manic attacks and exhaustion. Fatal doses depends on the atropine content, asphyxiation can occur with 100 mg of atropine which corresponds to 5 to 50 grams of belladonna. Please realize that the homeopathic dosage is very tiny and is not toxic.

Bryonia Alba

Bryonia alba, also known called white bryony and wild hops, is a perennial found in Europe and England. This is another plant that is extremely poisonous. If an accidental poisoning occurs, it can cause violent vomiting, extreme inflammation and diarrhea, leading to death usually in a matter of hours. Bryonia has displayed antitumoral effects, acts as a purgative and can have a strong hypoglycemic affect.

Conditions in which bryonia is used include acute and chronic infectious diseases, backache, body aches, cough, diarrhea, diuretic, dizziness, emetic, fatigue, fever, flu, gastrointestinal disorders, headache, joint pain, liver disorders, lumbago, metabolic disorders, migraine headache, pain from broken bones, respiratory tract disorders, rheumatism and sore throat.

Precautions: This drug is highly toxic when freshly harvested. Over dosage can cause vomiting, bloody diarrhea, colic, kidney irritation, paralysis, collapse, and in some conditions, even death. Bryonia administered in homeopathic doses is considered safe for use.

Buttercup

Buttercup, scientifically known as *Ranunculus acris* and *bulbosus*, indigenous to northern Europe and the United States. The different types of the buttercup family have been medicinally in folk medicine for neuralgia and rheumatism.

Conditions in which buttercup is used include blisters, bronchitis, chronic skin conditions, gout, headaches, influenza, meningitis, neuralgia (especially intercostal neuralgia and herpes zoster), pleural pain and rheumatism.

Precautions: Not to be taken during pregnancy. Extended use topically can cause blistering to the skin that are difficult to heal. Internal usage can cause irritation to the gastrointestinal tract, colic and diarrhea. This usually only occurs with usage of freshly harvested plants. The homeopathic preparations are sate for use.

Causticum

Causticum is derived from a preparation made of caustic, slaked lime (calcium hydroxide) and potassium bisulphate. This particular remedy was invented by Dr. Hahnemann, the founder of homeopathy.

Conditions in which causticum is used include constipation, cough, cramps, cystitis, facial paralysis, indigestion, joint pain, laryngitis, muscle cramps and pain, rheumatism, sore throat, urinary incontinence and retention.

Precautions: Safe in homeopathic doses.

Cell Salts

Cell salts, also called "tissue salts," were discovered by Dr. W. H. Schuessler, M.D. in 1873. He isolated 12 mineral compounds which he called "cell salts." It was Dr. Schuessler's belief that if the body became deficient in any of these important minerals, an abnormal or disease condition could occur. He found that cell salts could be very effective in the treatment of various diseases and maladies. This was the beginning of Dr. Schuessler's "biochemic system of medicine." Over the intervening years, the biochemic theory concerning the use of minerals as therapy has become better understood and very helpful as a treatment modality. Dr. Schuessler believed that the 12 cell salts contained all the active ingredients used by traditional homeopathy. Because of this, I have included the cell salts in the homeopathic section.

All of the cell salts have value in the treatment of pain, both as singular remedies and in combination. Cell salts can be useful as an antispasmodic, for arthritis, back pain, bruises, bursitis, burns, cancer, coccyx pain, colic, cramps, ear pain, eye pain, face pain, foot pain, gout, growing pain, head pain, headaches, heart pain, injuries, joint(s) pain, leg pain, low back pain, menstrual pain, migraine headaches, muscular pain, neck pain, nerve pain, neuralgia, rheumatoid arthritis, sciatica, sprains and strains, stomach ache, teeth and trauma pain. In addition to the pain syndromes, cell salts can be used to treat practically every type of disease. Cell salts deserve serious study and attention. In my practice, I have utilized them in difficult cases with excellent results. For further information, see the Recommended Reading List at the end of this book.

The following are the 12 cell salts, including their abbreviations, and an example of a pain syndrome that they can help resolve.

Cell Salt Name:	Pain Syndrome
Calc Fluor – Calcium Fluoride	Leg pain, Poor circulation
Calc Phos – Calcium Phosphate	Joint pain, Elbow & hip
Calc Sulph – Calcium Sulphate	Headache
Ferr Phos – Ferrum Phosphate	Neuralgia, Intercostal
Kali Mur – Potassium Chloride	Back pain
Kali Phos – Potassium Phosphate	Breast pain
Kali Sulph – Potassium Sulfate	Rheumatoid Arthritis pain
Mag Phos – Magnesium Phosphate	Muscle cramping pain
Nat Mur – Sodium Chloride	Arthritis pain
Nat Phos – Sodium Phosphate	Knee pain
Nat Sulph – Sodium Sulphate	Coccyx pain
Silica – Silica Oxide	Foot pain

Cell salts can provide a valuable form of treatment, both as a first line approach and in an adjunct capacity.

Herb Paris

Herb paris, known scientifically as *Paris quadrifolia*, is indigenous to Europe and parts of Russia. This plant, also called "one berry," is another plant which is poisonous. There have been documented incidents over a century ago in which children were poisoned after mistakenly eating the fruit of Herb Paris, thinking that it was blueberries.

Herb Paris is helpful for headaches, migraines, neuralgia, nervous tension, dizziness, palpitations.

Precautions: This drug is considered poisonous. Symptoms of poisoning, after ingesting the berries, include nausea, vomiting, diarrhea, miosis (contraction of the eye pupil) and headache. In homeopathic dosages, it is safe.

Monk's-Hood

Monk's-Hood, known scientifically as *Aconitum napellus,* grows in Europe, Russian and central Asia. It contains the chemical substance "aconite," which is a deadly poison. This potent poison has been used in times past for hunting and by assassins. In homeopathic medicine it has proven very valuable for fevers and inflammations.

Conditions in which monk's-hood is used include arthritis, fever, gout, inflammation, migraine headaches, myalgia, muscular and articular rheumatism, neuralgia (especially trigeminal and intercostal types), pain, pleurisy and skin inflammations.

Precautions: Monk's-Hood is highly toxic and extremely poisonous. With the exception of homeopathic preparations, administration of this drug is prohibited. Because of its potential for harm, use only under the care of a homeopathic physician.

Pulsatilla

The pulsatilla plant is part of the Ranunclulaceae family and goes by a number of different names: Meadow anemone, pasque flower and wind flower. This is a perennial plant that grows in many parts of Europe. In ancient times, the pulsatilla plant was used extensively for a wide variety of maladies, especially inflammations and ulcers. It has a number of wide ranging actions and has been called the "Queen of Homeopathic Remedies."

Conditions in which pulsatilla can be useful include back pain, bronchitis, constipation, cough, dyspepsia, earache, eye inflammation, fever, flatulence (gas), gastric upset, headache, hayfever, indigestion, insomnia, joint pain, labor pain, migraine headache, neuralgia, painful menstruation, pharyngitis, sciatica, sore throat, teething, toothache and varicose veins.

Precautions: Not to be taken during pregnancy.

Yellow Jessamine

Yellow jessamine, known scientifically as *Gelsemium sempervirens*, is a climbing plant found in the southern United States. Gelsemium is poisonous in large dose. It has vasodilatory, hypotensive and bronchodilatory effects.

Conditions in which yellow jessamine are used include fever, gastric disorders, headaches, heartburn, inflammation, influenza, migraine headaches and neuralgia. It has also been used for infectious states.

Precautions: With proper administration of homeopathic doses, no adverse reactions are likely. Possible side effects from overdose can include heaviness of the eyelids, double vision, difficulty moving the eyeball, dryness of the mouth and vomiting. Potential poisoning through over dosage exists, so caution should be taken.

Topicals

Natural medicine has a long history of using natural substances externally on the body for a variety of maladies. This has been especially true of "folk medicine" and folklore over the centuries. Many cultures worldwide have examples and remedies that use plants and herbs topically, typically with excellent results.

This section will discuss ten different substances that can be used as topical agents. With exception of DMSO, all are "natural" substances. DMSO has been included in this this book because it has amazing therapeutic properties. Some of the substances have been discussed previously in other sections. If this is the case, a notation is made to refer to that specific section for further information.

Arnica

For the general information on Arnica, please see its listing in the Herbal Section.

Arnica is an excellent topical that can be used for a number of conditions externally. As noted previously, Arnica has been used in both herbal and homeopathic preparations for its analgesic and anti-inflammatory effects.

Conditions that Arnica can be used topically for include: Arthritis, blunt trauma, bruises, contusions, inflammatory conditions of the skin, muscle and joints, joint pain.

Precautions: Topically, Arnica has no known negative qualities.

Calendula

The scientific name for Calendula is *Calendula Officinalis*. It is commonly known as Marigold. Calendula is grown in Europe, Asia and in the United States but has almost worldwide distribution. Folklore uses of Calendula date back literally centuries. Calendula has antimicrobial, antifungal, antibacterial, antiviral, antiphlogistic (inflammation reducing) and vulnerary (wound healing) actions. It has a stimulating effect on the immune system, inhibit tumors and can have an inhibitory effect on the central nervous system. It has been used as a topical agent for a variety of conditions, especially to promote wound healing and reduce inflammation.

Conditions that Calendula is used for topically include antifungal, bee stings, burns, dry skin, eczema, inflammation (of muscles, joints and skin), muscle pain, sunburn and wound healing.

Precautions: Essentially none from topical usage. There is a low potential for skin sensitization with frequent usage.

Cayenne

For general information on Cayenne, please see its listing in the Herbal Section.

As previously noted, Cayenne has been used medicinally for centuries. In regard to its topical usage, the chief chemical compound, capsaicin, has proven to be very effective for a variety of conditions.

Conditions in which Cayenne can be used externally as a topical agent include arm and spine pain, arthritis, chronic low back pain, frostbite, joint pain, muscle pain, muscle spasms, rheumatic conditions

and sore throats. Side effects: Blistering to skin, allergic reaction to skin and burning from being placed
accidently in sensitive areas such as the eyes.

Precautions: Potential side effects with topical
use can include allergic skin reactions, blistering of the
skin and burning if the cayenne is accidently placed in
sensitive areas such as the eyes.

Cloves

Cloves have a long history of medicinal use that
continues through this day. Perhaps the main component of cloves is the oil that is extracted from its flower
buds and fruit. Cloves have a distinct smell and taste,
one you won't forget once you have experienced it. It is
used as an antibacterial, antifungal, antihistamine,
antiseptic and antispasmodic. Cloves are best used as
a topical agent for its analgesic properties.

Conditions in which Cloves can be used externally as a topical agent include antiseptic, dental analgesic, fungal infections, inflammation of skin and
mucous membranes, local anesthetic, muscular pain
relief, ringworm infections, skin antibacterial and
toothaches.

Precautions: Caution should be taken when
using Clove oil on mucous membranes as it can be an
irritant.

DMSO

DMSO is an amazing substance, even though it
is not specifically considered a "natural" one. DMSO,
chemically known as dimethylglycine, is a by-product

of wood processing in paper manufacturing. It is an oily substance with a garlic-like odor. It is an excellent solvent and has found many commercial uses in this capacity in industrial settings. It is widely used in antifreeze, paint thinners and as a degreaser. For all of this "industrial" capability, DMSO also has incredible value as a therapeutic agent in the treatment of a variety of maladies. DMSO is traditionally used topically, although it can be administered intravenously by a doctor specializing in its use. DMSO is very rapidly absorbed through the skin and into the bloodstream. A common side effect with DMSO use is the "taste" of it within the mouth that is experienced soon after applying topically.

Conditions in which DMSO has be used externally as a topical agent include acne, arthritis (osteroarthritis, rheumatoid arthritis and other arthritic variants), back pain, blunt trauma, bone pain, burns, cancer, contusions, headaches, herpes, keloids (scars), joint pain, musculoskeletal problems (including spinal, pelvic, extremity, joint, muscular injuries and pain), sciatica, sinusitis (placed topically just inside the nostrils), skin ulcers, sports injuries, sprains and strains. DMSO may also have potential usages for cystitis, infections, mental disabilities, neurological disorders, scleroderma and urinary problems.

Precautions: This product should never be taken orally. It should not be used by children. Intravenous administration should only be performed by a qualified doctor and with caution.

Eucalyptus

Eucalyptus, scientifically known as eucalyptus globulus, is another one of those substances that has a history of usage that extends back literally centuries. It can be used both internally and externally for a variety of ailments. The chief component of eucalyptus is a volatile oil which contains the chemical cineole. It is grown in many subtropical areas of the world including Europe, Africa, Asia and America.

Conditions in which eucalyptus can be used externally as a topical agent include anti-inflammatory, antiseptic, arthritis, asthma, bronchitis, coughs, joint pain, muscle pain, neuralgia, rheumatoid arthritis, sinusitis and wound healing.

Precautions: Use caution if using eucalyptus oil on infants and small children. Avoid application to the face as it may cause a glottal or bronchial spasm leading to asphyxiation.

Garlic

Garlic, scientifically known as *Allium sativum*, is a well known and popular perennial that is cultivated worldwide. Garlic has many used, both medicinally and nutritionally. One of the main substances, within garlic that is believed to be responsible for its pharmacological activity is chemical "allicin." Garlic is known for its positive effects on atherosclerosis, high blood pressure and high cholesterol. Externally, garlic has been used for a wide variety of ailments in folk medicine including muscle pain, neuralgia, corns and warts.

Conditions in which garlic can be used externally as a topical agent include antibacterial activity, antifungal, anti-inflammatory, antiseptic, arthritis, muscle pain, neuralgia, otitis media, rheumatoid arthritis and sciatica.

Precautions: On rare occasions, frequent topical applications may lead to allergic skin reaction.

Lavender

Lavender, scientifically known as *Lavandula spp.*, has many different species within its family. Lavender has a long history of use in folk medicine, being a popular remedy for a wide range of conditions. It is considered an anti-spasmodic, circulatory stimulant, general tonic, antibacterial, analgesic, carminative and antiseptic. Topically, lavender is applied as a liquid from a decoction or oil.

Lavender can be used externally as a topical agent for arthritis, asthma, bronchial spasm, cough, eczema, headaches, insect bites and stings, joint pain, migraine headache, muscle pain, muscle spasms, neualgia, rheumatism and sunburns.

Precautions: Essentially none for topical usage.

Peppermint

Peppermint is a well known perennial cultivated in Europe and the United States and is scientifically known as Mentha piperita. Peppermint has a long tradition of use in both Eastern and Western natural medicine, in which both the plant and its oil have been utilized. It is considered an antibacterial, antispasmodic, antiseptic and has carmative effects. It has been used for a variety of gastrointestinal disorders (nausea, indigestion, heartburn, etc.), colds, flu, sore throats, toothaches and cramps. The volatile oil, especially with topical use, has been found to have localized analgesic properties. It is very complex, with more than 100 chemical compounds found within it. The primary component is menthol and its derivatives.

Peppermint can be used externally as a topical agent for arthritis, asthma, bronchitis, cough, fever, headaches, inflammation (joints, muscle and skin), itching, joint pain, menstrual pain, muscle pain, muscle spasms, neuralgia and rheumatism.

Precautions: Use caution if using eucalyptus oil on infants and small children. Avoid application to the face as it may cause a glottal or bronchial spasm leading to asphyxiation.

Wintergreen

Wintergreen is another of the perennial plants which is scientifically known as *Gaultheria procumbens.* It is indigenous to North America and Canada. Wintergreen and its volatile oil have been used both internally and externally for a variety of ailments. It is considered a carmative, tonic and antiseptic. The main chemical component is methyl salicylate, which is structurally similar to aspirin. This helps explain the volatile oil's analgesic properties.

Wintergreen can be used externally as a topical agent for arthritis, asthma, bronchitis, cough, fever, headaches, inflammation (joints, muscle and skin), itching, joint pain, menstrual pain, muscle pain, muscle spasms, neuralgia, pleurisy, rheumatism, sciatica.

Precautions: Potential for contact allergies exists with topical administration.

There are dozens of other natural substances that can be used topically to treat pain directly or some aspect of pain causing conditions. Examples include black pepper, chondroitin sulfate, glucosamine sulfate, Japanese mint, larch, MSM, onion, scotch pine and spruce. All substances that can be used topically to address pain should be evaluated and integrated in to a pain management program.

Module Two:

Natural Physical Methods

There are many physical approaches to pain relief. Included in this group are Acupuncture, Chiropractic, Exercise and Stretching, Massage Therapy, and Physical Therapy. This is not an all-inclusive list by any means. Other physical approaches include Cranialsacral Therapy, Meditation and Relaxation Techniques, Osteopathy, Yoga and others. To adequately and fully discuss each of these approaches would require much more room than is available in this book. The information for each of these subjects can easily fill multiple books and in fact does. There are many excellent books available which cover and discuss these approaches in-depth. I highly recommend that you read and study those topics here which interest you. In regard to pain relief, by themselves and as part of an overall pain relief program; all of these approaches have outstanding benefits the should not be ignored.

Because of the limits of space, these physical approaches will only be introduced to you in the same manner as the other sections of this book.

Acupuncture

Acupuncture had its origins in China and has been practiced for over five thousand years. This unique health approach is based on the belief that health is determined by balancing "Qi" (also called Chi). Qi is believed to be the vital energy of all life.

Acupuncturist believe that qi circulates in the body along twelve "major" energy pathways which they call "meridians." These meridians are linked to major organs and organ systems. Within these meridians are literally thousands of "acupuncture points" that are utilized by acupuncturists to balance and effect the flow of qi. It is believed that qi energy flow becomes unbalanced with disease states and other maladies. To effect and improve health, accupuncturist's manipulate qi through the use of acupuncture needles and non-needle applications to the acupuncture points. Acupuncture needles are thin, specialized needles which are inserted under the skin into these acupuncture points. It has been documented that acupuncture can relieve and decrease pain and help in a variety of health conditions. Pain is an area that acupuncture has proven to be very successful in relieving. It appears that acupuncture stimulates the release of endorphins and enkaphalins, which are the body's natural pain relieving substances (see Section One: Pain mechanisms and pathways).

Conditions in which acupuncture can be used include addictions, arthritis, asthma, bronchitis, cough, fever, fibromyalgia, headaches, inflammation (joints, muscle and skin), itching, joint pain, menstrual pain, mental disorders, migraine headaches, muscle pain, muscle spasms, neuralgia, pain syndromes, pleurisy, rheumatism,sciatica and tennis elbow. Please note that I have focused more on pain related conditions here. Acupuncture, especially in traditional eastern medicine, is used to treat most diseases and conditions including the common cold, duodenal ulcer, Meniere's disease, myopia, sinusitis, stroke and its related symptoms, etc.

Precautions: Potential for skin reactions from the needles can occur, but is considered rare.

Chiropractic

Chiropractic is a natural, drug free approach to health care that is based on the body's innate, built-in ability to heal itself. This "innate" intelligence within the body is basic to our capability to heal ourselves from a variety of everyday stresses, maladies and health problems. Chiropractic utilizes "adjustments" of the spine and joints to influence the nervous system, and through this, the body's innate intelligence and various natural defense mechanisms for healing. The chiropractic adjustment is performed by the hands or using specialized adjusting instruments and actually "moves and manipulates" the spine. This is very important because the spinal column and spinal cord coordinates and controls the functions of all the systems in the body. Misalignments of the spine, called "subluxations" of the spine by chiropractors, creates blockages and nerve interference which in turn cause pain and reduce the body's normal capacity for healing. Chiropractic adjustments return the spine to normal alignment which essential for optimum health and function.

Conditions in which chiropractic can be used include arthritis, asthma, back pain, fibromyalgia, frozen shoulder, headaches, inflammation (joints, muscle and skin), joint pain (both in the spine and extremities), low back pain, menstrual pain, migraine headaches, muscle pain, muscle spasms, neck pain, neuralgia, pain syndromes, pleurisy, rheumatism, sciatica and scoliosis. ***Please note that I have focused more on pain related conditions here. Chiropractic can be used to treat a variety of diseases and conditions including addictions, bedwetting, constipation, gynecological disorders, otitis media, tinnitus, etc..

Precautions: Potential for muscular reactions, such as muscle spasm, can occur occasionally following a chiropractic adjustment. Chiropractic adjustments are contraindicated with bone tumors, fractures, certain types of cancer and severe osteoporosis.

Exercise and Stretching

It has been understood for ages that movement of the body has inherent health benefits. This basic concept has been greatly expanded as our knowledge of the body has grown; especially in regard to physical function, the mind/body connection and the body's basic health needs. There are multiple positive benefits to exercising and stretching the body. These encompass all aspects of our being; including the physical, mental, emotional and spiritual.

Exercise and stretching from the perspective of achieving pain relief must go beyond the general concepts of basic working out or performing a few toe touches each day. At this level, we consider exercise and stretching from a "therapeutic" aspect. Therapeutic exercise and stretching is based on the ultimate goal of achieving symptom-free movement and function. When we say "therapeutic," we are describing a program that is designed to facilitate a return to health as well as resolve the pain issues involved. It is an integrated program with multiple levels; from beginning basic movements that progressively increase to a person's end tolerance and capability. A therapeutic exercise and stretching program increases range of motion, flexibility, joint motion, muscle tone, muscle loading capacity and other variables. By positively impacting these components, we can in turn decrease and resolve pain, facilitate general health and impact a disease process.

Typically, therapeutic exercise and stretching programs are prepared and set up by a health care professional who monitors your progress. If your pain is from a disease process or other health condition, it becomes critical that you have the expertise of a professional to design, monitor and alter your program as needed. This is especially important in regard to symptoms and pain syndromes. An inappropriate program may not only make your pain worse but may cause your disease or condition to progress. I put in these warnings simply because I have seen the unfortunate results of poorly designed therapeutic programs.

Conditions in which exercise and stretching can be used include arthritis, back pain, fibromyalgia, frozen shoulder, headaches, joint pain (both in the spine and extremities), low back pain, menstrual pain, migraine headaches, muscle pain, muscle spasms, neck pain, neuralgia, pain syndromes, rheumatism, sciatica, sprain, strains and scoliosis. ***Please note that I have focused more on pain related conditions here. Exercise and stretching can be used to treat a variety of diseases and conditions including depression and other mental disorders, neurological disorders, pregnancy, pulmonary conditions, respiratory conditions, stress relief, stroke rehabilitation, vascular disorders and weight control.

Precautions: Potential for muscular reactions, such as muscle spasm or inflammation, can occur if exercise and/or stretching is performed too aggressively or advanced to quickly. Exercise and stretching can be contraindicated with certain diseases and conditions. Please consult a health care professional for information in this regard.

Massage Therapy

Massage has been used in some form for literally thousands of years. The "laying on of hands," especially by rubbing, has been a traditional form of healing used by many cultures. Massage was used by the ancient Greeks and Romans as a principle means of healing as well as pain relief.

There a variety of massage therapy versions, from basic gentle stroking to shiatsu (pressure pointing). All have value through touch and muscle manipulation. Certainly, pain relief is at the forefront of this value from a therapeutic standpoint. Massage therapy can have many positive effects beyond that of pain relief, including as a stress reliever, for circulation problems, depression, etc.

Conditions in which massage can be used include anxiety, arthritis, back pain, bronchial congestion, cancer, circulation problems, colds, congestion, depression, fibromyalgia, frozen shoulder, headaches, heart disorders, high blood pressure, hyperactivity, insomnia, joint pain (both in the spine and extremities), low back pain, menstrual pain, migraine headaches, muscle pain, muscle spasms, neck pain, neuralgia, pain syndromes, rheumatism, sciatica, sinusitis, sprain, strains, stress and tension. ***Please note that massage can have a positive impact on many diseases and conditions. Including a variety of mental disorders, neurological disorders, pregnancy, pulmonary conditions, respiratory conditions and vascular disorders.

Precautions: Massage is contraindicated with skin eruptions (boils, rashes, scabies, etc..), bruises, varicose veins, fever, inflamed joints, tumors, undiagnosed lumps, thrombosis and phlebitis (unless under a doctor's supervision).

Physical Therapy

Physical therapy is a general term which is used to describe a number of approaches to pain relief, rehabilitation and general health. Within this group we are interested in a number of physical modalities including ice (cryotherapy), heat (dry and moist types), hydrotherapy (water therapy – i.e. jacuzzi), electrical muscle stimulation, tens, traction and ultrasound. A brief description of each of these follows.

Ice (cryotherapy): This therapy utilizes cold as a therapeutic approach. By placing cold over the involved area, we can sedate nerves, reduce muscular spasms, reduce inflammation and decrease pain. Icing types include cold/ice packs, frozen water and immersion therapy in ice water.

Heat: There are two type of heat that are typically used. The first is dry heat, such as is obtained from a heating pad. The other type is moist heat which can be obtained from a moist hot pack or heat-moistened towel. By placing heat over the involved area, we decrease muscle spasms, reduce muscle tightness and decrease pain.

Hydrotherapy: This is basically water therapy and can involve heated or cold water. An example of the heated type would be a jacuzzi. The cold water version typically is a cold bath. Both of these types can also be done through a shower. These therapies can be used to effect a localized area or for full body therapy. The effects of these therapies are the same as those listed for ice and heat.

Electrical Muscle Stimulation: These modalities are machine based with pads placed over the involved areas of the body; typically soft tissue (muscle). These machines put an electrical current at therapeutic levels into the soft tissue to stimulate a response, i.e. on a muscle will cause that muscle to contract at a prescribed rate or at a constant contraction. The point of this therapy is to cause the muscle to contract, then relax. This type of therapy is to reduce and decrease muscular spasm, hypertonicity and spasm, decrease inflammation and reduce soft tissue adhesions. These machines are also used in a rehabilitative capacity to work weakened or atrophied muscles.

Tens (aka: Transcutaneous electrical nerve stimulation): This therapy also involves applying an electrical current to affected nerves, only at a micro level. Tens machines are used for pain control by causing nerve conduction to be blocked and reducing nerve irritation. It is believed that Tens units also stimulate the production of endorphins, the body's natural painkillers.

Traction: There are two types of traction – intermittent and constant. These types of therapies can be performed on specialized machines or by hand. The purpose of this therapy is stretch effect muscles and soft tissue, reducing muscle spasms, hypertonicity and tightness. It is also used to open up spinal units to take pressure of the intervertebral discs and spinal nerves.

Ultrasound: This machine-based therapy takes an electrical current and translates it through a soundhead with a specialized crystal which turns the current into mechanical sound waves. This soundhead is used over the affected areas, utilizing a coupling agent to transmit the sound waves through the skin. It is used to reduce inflammation, muscular spasms, muscle tightness, pain relief, organization of new scar tissue, breakdown of old scar tissue and adhesions.

Each of these physical therapy modalities has excellent value for pain relief and in addressing a variety of conditions. They can be applied as both home based therapy and as an in-office therapeutic approach by health care professionals. I have found them to be an excellent adjunct to my treatment programs for their pain relieving capabilities.

Precautions: For those modalities which are machine based and of a commercial grade, it is imperative that their application be performed by a qualified health care professional who is trained in their operation and clinical uses. These machines can burn tissue, cause inflammatory responses, cause muscular spasms, cause frostbite and cause and increase pain. Always use caution when using physical therapy modalities and make sure you fully understand their application and usage.

---

*This **Quick Access Chart** beginning on the following page has been provided to give you immediate information in regard to effecting 50 different common pain-related syndromes. For quick pain relieving methods, look up your specific problem and go to the category called "Immediate Pain Relief." For specifically working on the underlying condition to relieve pain, go to the category called "Secondary Pain Relieving Methods."*

When using this chart keep in mind that there are many reasons a disease process or condition may arise. Your particular problem may require a different set of natural treatment approaches which has not been listed. This is not all-inclusive. There are literally hundreds of other diseases and conditions which did not make this book simply because of necessary space. Many of them can be approached naturally with excellent results.

Important Caution: *For all the conditions listed, it is critical that they be properly diagnosed and their causes determined. This almost always requires the assistance of a health care professional. Without the correct information, any treatment program may well prove to be ineffective or even worse, could be potentially harmful.*

Module Three:
Pain Resolving Strategies

COMPLAINT	IMMEDIATE RELIEF	SECONDARY RELIEF

ABDOMEN, ORGANS & THE DIGESTIVE SYSTEM:

COMPLAINT	IMMEDIATE RELIEF	SECONDARY RELIEF
Constipation	**1. Water:** Drink 6-8 8 oz glasses in 24 hours. **2. Aloe Vera Juice:** Drink 2 ozs 3 times in 24 hours. **3. Cascara Sagrada:** 2 caps 3 times /day with food. **4. Homeopathy:** Nux vomica 12c dose, 3-4 pellets under the tongue sublingually 2-3 times day. **5. Psyllium Husk and Seed:** 1 to 2 tbs in 8 ozs of water 2-3 times /day.	**1. Exercise:** Walk briskly at least 1 mile /day, abdominal workout (low impact sit-ups and crunches to the abdomen with the shoulders remaining close to the ground, chin to chest - squeeze/contract the abdominal muscles; leg raises). **2. Chiropractic Adjustments:** Low back, pelvic and sacroiliac. Initially may need 2-3 visits /week for 4 weeks. **3. Fiber:** Eat at at least 3 fiber sources /day. Eat a high fiber diet. **4.** Eliminate all causes of constipation. **5. Herbals:** Use 1 of these only when needed, not daily. Fennel:1-2 caps 2 times /day or drink a 6 oz cup of tea steeped for 5 min. 2 times /day. Alfalfa: 1-2 caps 2 times /day. Rhubarb: 1-2 caps 2 times /day. Senna: 1-2 caps 2 times /day. For combination formulas: Use as directed.
Gallstones	**1. Fasting:** Fast on water or juice (carrot/apple/cucumber) up to 3 days. Drink 6-8 ozs morning, mid-morning, noon, mid-afternoon and evening. **2. Gallbladder Flush:** Can be done in conjunction with the fast above with caution. First Day – One 8 oz glass of fresh apple juice at 8 am; then 2 glasses at 10 am, noon, 2 pm, 4 pm and then 6 pm. Day Two – Same as the first day Plus: At bedtime, take 2-4 ozs of olive oil in 1 8 oz glass of warm water and with one 6-8 oz glass of lemon or apple juice. Perform for only 2 days. **3. Aloe Vera:** Drink aloe vera juice, 2 ozs 4 times /day for 24 hours. **4. Castor Oil/Herbal Pack:** Make a castor oil pack and include burdock root, slippery elm and thyme and place over the right abdomen. **5. Peppermint:** Drink tea 6 ozs steeped for 5 min. 3 times a day or take 3-5 drops of oil 5 times a day.	**1.** Decrease fat intake in the diet. Replace with the "good fats," from such sources as flaxseed oil, fish oil or primrose oil. Take 2 softgels /day for flaxseed and primrose oil. For fish oil, take 2 tbs/day. **2.** Eliminate any food allergies. **3. Multi-Enzyme:** Take 1 with each meal; at least 3 /day. **4. Acidophilus/Lactobacillus:** Take 1 tbs 2-3 times /day approximately 30 minutes prior to a meal. Alternative: Take 1-2 caps 2-3 times /day approximately 30 minutes prior to a meal. **5.** Avoid animal products.

COMPLAINT	IMMEDIATE RELIEF	SECONDARY RELIEF
Gastritis	**1. Herbal combination:** Create a tea with licorice root, slippery elm, marshmallow, echinacea, goldenseal and pau de arco. Mix 1 part of each (bulk herb) in 10 ozs of water, steep 10 minutes, cool. Drink one 6 oz cup every 4-6 hours, up to 4 in the first 24 hours. **2. Chamomile:** Take 1-2 caps initially; then take 1-2 caps twice more during first 24 hours. Alternative: Can make a tea by steeping for 5-10 minutes. Drink 6 oz cup 3 times /day first 24 hours. **3. Homeopathy:** Ferr Phos (Iron Phosphate) and Kali Mur (Potassium Chloride). Use 6c to 12c versions. Take 4 tabs under the tongue sublinqually. Repeat each hour for first 3 hours, then every 3-4 hours thereafter; for the first 24 hours.	**1. Vitamin C:** Use a calcium or potassium ascorbate form (buffered). Take up to bowel tolerance (so does not cause diarrhea). If you are currently not taking vitamin C, begin with one 500 mg /day. Each week, raise this level by 500 mg until bowel tolerance is reached. On average, a dose of 3000 to 5000 mg /day is what will be needed. **2. Multiple Vitamin/Mineral:** Take 1-2 caps or softgels /day. (moderate dose- look at the B vitamins - should be at least 25 mg up to 50 mg for the 1-2 cap/softgel dose. Preference is a softgel form. **3. Zinc/Quercetin/Boswellia:** Take up to 50 mg of zinc /day until gastritis is under control; for quercetin and boswellia, take 2 caps 2 times /day. **4. Stress Relief:** Massage Therapy: 1/2 to 1 hour, full body; meditation (10-15 min.) in quiet room, comfortable position, counting and controlling breathing), muscular relaxation technique (lying on the bed or floor, begin with toes, contracting then relaxing each muscle group in the body as you work up to the head, focus on your breathing, repeat twice); exercise (at least 20-30 minutes, aerobic, walking, bicycling, weight training, etc). **5. Build the immune system:** Eat a healthy, balanced high fiber diet, Use Supplements (including those mentioned already) plus additional vitamin A, beta-carotene, calcium, magnesium, potassium, etc. and herbs such as elderberry and cat's claw.
Heartburn & Gas Pain	**1. Charcoal:** Take 1-2 caps immediately; then take 2 caps twice more in the initial 24 hour period. **2. Ginger/Peppermint:** Take 2 caps immediately; then take 2 caps twice more in the initial 24 hour period. Alternative: Drink 6 ozs of combination tea, steep 5-10 min; drink 3 cups /day. **3. Multi-Enzyme:** Take a multi-enzyme complex 1-2 caps immediately; then take 1-2 twice more within the initial 24 hour period with food. **4. Papaya:** Chew 2 tabs every 4-6 hours.	**1. Fiber:** Increase fiber in diet by integrating whole grains, more fruits and vegetables etc. Make sure to get at least 3 fiber sources in /day. **2. Water:** Drink 6-8 8 oz glasses daily **3. Alfalfa:** Take 1-2 caps 2 times /day. **4. Eat slowly** and chew foods well; do not drink liquids with meals, don't eat when upset or stressed. **5. Vitamin B Complex:** 50 mg /day.

COMPLAINT	IMMEDIATE RELIEF	SECONDARY RELIEF
Irritable Bowel Syndrome (aka: Spastic Colon)	**1. Fiber:** Increase fiber in diet by integrating whole grains, more fruits and vegetables etc. Make sure to get at least 3 fiber sources in daily. **2. Water:** Drink 6-8 8 oz glasses daily. **3. Alfalfa:** Take 1-2 caps 2 times /day. **4. Eat slowly and chew foods well;** do not drink liquids with meals, don't eat when upset or stressed. **5. Vitamin B Complex:** 50 mg B vitamin complex 1 time/day.	**1. Fiber:** Increase fiber in diet by integrating whole grains, more fruits and vegetables etc. Make sure to get at least 3 fiber sources in cap/day. **2. Stress Relief:** (See number 4 under Gastritis). Perform each day. **3. Water:** Drink 6-8 8 oz glasses every day. **3. Alfalfa:** Take 1-2 caps 2 times /day. **4. Herbs:** Fennel: 1-2 caps 2 times /day; Wormwood: 1-2 caps 2 times /day.
Ulcers	**1. Aloe Vera:** Drink aloe vera juice, 2 ozs 4 times /day for 24 hours. **2. Ginger:** Take 2 caps immediately; then take 2 caps twice more in the initial 24 hour period. Alternative: Drink 6 ozs of ginger tea, steeped 5-10 minutes; drink 3-4 cups in initial 24 hour period. **3. Herbal combination:** Take 1 part each of deglycyrrhized licorice, chamomile, marshmallow and slippery elm; make a tea by steeping for 10 minutes and drinking 6 ozs immediately, followed by 2 additional cups in the 24 hour period. **4. Homeopathy:** Cell salts: Nat Phos (Sodium Phosphate) 3-4 pellets under tongue (sublingual) immediately; then every 2-3 hours for first 24 hours.	**1. Supplements:** Take 1-2 moderate level multiple vitamin/mineral daily. Take additional vitamin A, 1 cap 10,000-15,000 IU cap/day; zinc, one 30-40 mg cap cap/day; glutamine, 1 cap 500 mg 1-2 times /day. **2. Quercetin:** 2 caps 2 times /day. **3. Herbal Combination:** As listed above with deglycyrrhized licorice, chamomile, marshmallow and slippery elm. Drink two 6 oz cups/day of warm tea. **4. Vitamin E:** 400-800 IU cap/day. **5. Fiber:** Increase fiber in diet by integrating whole grains, more fruits and vegetables etc. Make sure to get at least 3 fiber sources in cap/day. Alternative: Psyllium seed and husk: 2 tbs in 8 ozs of water 2 times /day. Alternate this with whole foods.

BACK & NECK

Back Pain	**1. Ice:** Apply a pliable ice pack to the effected area. Place a paper towel or thin cloth between the skin and the ice pack. Ice for 20 minutes at a time. Can repeat 20 minutes every hour or every other hour in first 24 hours. **2. Chiropractic:** Have the effected area evaluated and adjusted by a chiropractor. Follow any instructions they may give in regard to the adjustment and adjunct care. **3. White willow bark:** Take 1-2 caps 3 times /day in first 24 hours. *Caution: If you have a history of ulcers or other gastrointestinal disorder which precludes you from taking aspirin, do not take this substance.* **4. Bromelain:** Take 2 caps 3 times /day in first 24 hours. **5. Herbal Combination:** Valerian, hops and skullcap: 2 caps 3 times /day	**1. Chiropractic:** Continue chiropractic adjustments. May need 2-3 per week for period of time. **2. Topically:** Apply arnica montana cream over effected area. Repeat 4-5 times in initial 24 hours. Alternative: Apply wintergreen oil or peppermint oil over effected area with same dosage. **3. Stretching:** Begin on day 3 after beginning of pain if tolerated; begin simple, gentle stretches to back. Lie on floor and tilt side-to-side, flatten low back against floor, squeeze shoulder blades together, etc. Perform 10 repetitions and/or hold each movement for a count of 10 and repeat twice each day. **4. Calcium and magnesium combo:** Take 3-4 softgels/caps each day with food in divided doses. Get at least 750-1,000 mg of calcium and 400-500

COMPLAINT	IMMEDIATE RELIEF	SECONDARY RELIEF
Back Pain Cont.	in first 24 hours. Alternative: Drink herbal tea combination of chamomile, lemon balm and passionflower; one part of each steeped in 6-8 ozs of water for 10 minutes, drink 3 cups /day.	mg of magnesium. **5. Massage Therapy:** Have a 1/2 to full hour therapeutic massage to the both the effected area and the body as a whole.
Intervertebral Disc Disorders	**1. Ice:** Apply a pliable ice pack to the effected area. Place a paper towel or thin cloth between the skin and the ice pack. Ice for 20 minutes at a time. Can repeat 20 minutes every hour or every other hour in first 24 hours. **2. Chiropractic:** Have the effected area evaluated and adjusted by a chiropractor. May require specialized techniques for disc condition. Follow any instructions they may give in regard to the adjustment and adjunct care. **3. White willow bark:** Take 1-2 caps 3 times/day in first 24 hours. *Caution: If you have a history of ulcers or other gastrointestinal disorder which precludes you from taking aspirin, do not take this substance.* **4. Bromelain:** Take 2 caps 3 times /day in first 24 hours. **5. Herbal Combination:** Combine of valerian, hops and skullcap: 2 caps 3 times /day in first 24 hours. Alternative: Drink herbal tea combination of chamomile, lemon balm and passionflower; 1 part of each steeped in 6-8 ozs of water for 10 minutes, drink 3 cups/day.	**1. Chiropractic:** Continue chiropractic adjustments. May need 2-3 per week for period of time. **2. Physical Therapy:** Utilize ice, moist heat, muscle stimulation, ultrasound, etc. to effected regions. Ice and heat can be done at home, the other modalities will need to be performed by a health care professional. **3. Stretching / Traction:** Begin on day 3 after beginning of pain if tolerable; begin simple, gentle stretches to back. Perform 10 repetitions for each movement, holding for a count of 10, repeat twice. Movements are performed while lying on your back on the floor and stretching longitudinally; pointing your toes 1 direction and your arms over your head in the opposite direction. **4. Calcium and magnesium:** 3-4 softgels/caps each day with food in divided doses. Get at least 750-1,000 mg of calcium and 400-500 mg of magnesium. **5. Massage Therapy:** 1/2 to 1 hour therapeutic massage to the both the effected area and the body as a whole.
Ligament Sprain	**1. Ice:** Apply a pliable ice pack to the effected area. Place a paper towel or thin cloth between the skin and the ice pack. Ice for 20 minutes at a time. Can repeat 20 minutes every hour or every other hour in first 24 hours. **2.** If applicable, wrap effected area in an ace bandage firmly to apply compression and keep elevated. **3. White willow bark:** Take 1-2 caps 3 times /day in first 24 hours. Caution: If you have a history of ulcers or other gastrointestinal disorder which precludes you from taking aspirin, do not take. **4. Bromelain:** Take 2 caps 3 times a day in first 24 hours.	**1. B-complex:** 50-100 mg/day. **2. Vitamin C:** Use a calcium or potassium ascorbate form (buffered). Take up to bowel tolerance. If you are currently not taking vitamin C, begin with one 500 mg cap /day. Each week, raise this level by 500 mg until bowel tolerance is reached. Average dose: 3000 to 5000 mg /day. **3. Stretching:** Begin stretching/flexibility movements by day 2 or 3, depending on tolerance. Use abbreviated, gentle motions. Perform 10 repetitions and/or hold each movement for a count of 10 and repeat twice. Slowly increase amount of motion over time. **4. Exercise:** Over time, begin exercise program to effected area soft tissue. Depending on area impacted, this will

COMPLAINT	IMMEDIATE RELIEF	SECONDARY RELIEF
Ligament Sprain Cont.	**5. Topically:** Apply arnica montana cream over effected area. Repeat 4-5 times within initial 24 hours.	involve some type of progressive, resistance training.
Low Back Pain	**1. Ice:** Apply a pliable ice pack to the effected area. Place a paper towel or thin cloth between the skin and the ice pack. Ice for 20 minutes at a time. Repeat 20 minutes every hour or every other hour in first 24 hours. **2. Chiropractic:** Have the effected area evaluated and adjusted by a chiropractor. Follow any instructions they may give in regard to the adjustment and adjunct care. **3. White willow bark:** Take 1-2 caps 3 times /day in first 24 hours. Caution: If you have a history of ulcers or other gastrointestinal disorder which precludes you from taking aspirin, do not take. **4. Bromelain:** 2 caps 3 times/day in first 24 hours. **5. Herbal Combination:** Valerian, hops and skullcap: 2 caps 3 times /day in first 24 hours. Alternative: Drink herbal tea combination of chamomile, lemon balm and passionflower; 1 part of each steeped in 6-8 ozs of water for 10 minutes, drink 3 cups /day.	**1. Chiropractic:** Continue chiropractic adjustments. May need 2-3 per week for period of time. **2. Topically:** Apply arnica montana cream over effected area. Repeat 4-5 times within initial 24 hours. Alternative: Apply wintergreen oil or peppermint oil over effected area with same dosage. **3. Stretching:** Begin on day 3 after beginning of pain if tolerable; begin with simple, gentle stretches to the low back. Lie on your back on the floor. Bring each knee to the chest and hold; flatten the low back against floor; with knees bent and feet flat on floor, push pelvis toward ceiling; roll onto your side, bringing both knees up and roll top shoulder backwards; etc. Perform 10 repetitions and/or hold each movement for a count of 10 and repeat twice daily. **4. Calcium / Magnesium Combo:** Take 3-4 softgels/caps each day with food in divided doses. Get at least 750-1000 mg of calcium and 400-500 mg of magnesium. **5. Massage Therapy:** 1/2 hour to full hour therapeutic massage to the both the effected area and the body as a whole.
Muscular Injuries, And Strains	**1. Ice:** Apply a pliable ice pack to the effected area. Place a paper towel or thin cloth between the skin and the ice pack. Ice for 20 minutes at a time. Can repeat 20 minutes every hour or every other hour in first 24 hours. **2. Chiropractic:** Have the effected area evaluated and adjusted by a chiropractor. Follow any instructions they may give in regard to the adjustment and adjunct care. **3. Topically:** Apply arnica montana cream over effected area. Repeat 4-5 times within initial 24 hours. **4. Bromelain:** Take 2 caps 3 times /day in first 24 hours. **5. Herbal Combination:** Valerian, hops and skullcap: 2 caps 3 times /day in first 24 hours. Alternative:	**1. Chiropractic:** Continue chiropractic adjustments. May need 2-3 per week for period of time. **2. Topically:** Apply arnica montana cream over effected area. Repeat 4-5 times within initial 24 hours. Alternative: Apply wintergreen oil or peppermint oil over effected area with same dosage. **3. Stretching:** Begin on day 3 after beginning of pain if tolerated; begin simple, gentle stretches to back. Stretch the effected areas. Perform 10 repetitions or hold for count of 10 for each movement and repeat twice each day. **4. Calcium / magnesium combo:** Get at least 750-1000 mg of calcium and 400-500 mg of magnesium each day with food in divided doses. **5. Massage Therapy:** 1/2 to 1 hour therapeutic massage to the both the effected area and the body as a whole.

COMPLAINT	IMMEDIATE RELIEF	SECONDARY RELIEF
Muscular Injuries, And Strains Cont.	Drink herbal tea combination of chamomile, lemon balm and passionflower; one part of each steeped in 6-8 ozs of water for 10 minutes, drink 3 cups /day.	
Neck Pain	**1. Ice:** Apply a pliable ice pack to the effected area. Place a paper towel or thin cloth between the skin and the ice pack. Ice for 20 minutes at a time. Can repeat 20 minutes every hour or every other hour in first 24 hours. **2. Chiropractic:** Have the effected area evaluated and adjusted by a chiropractor. Follow any instructions they may give in regard to the adjustment and adjunct care. **3. White willow bark:** Take 1-2 caps 3 times /day in first 24 hours. Caution: If you have a history of ulcers or other gastrointestinal disorder which precludes you from taking aspirin, do not take this substance. **4. Bromelain:** Take 2 caps 3 times /day in first 24 hours. **5. Herbal Combination:** Valerian, hops and skullcap: 2 caps 3 times /day in first 24 hours. Alternative: Drink herbal tea combination of chamomile, lemon balm and passionflower; one part of each steeped in 6-8 ozs of water for 10 minutes, drink 3 cups /day.	**1. Chiropractic:** Continue chiropractic adjustments. May need 2-3 per week for period of time. **2. Topically:** Apply arnica montana cream over effected area. Repeat 4-5 times within initial 24 hours. Alternative: Apply wintergreen oil or peppermint oil over effected area with same dosage. **3. Stretching:** Begin on day 3 after beginning of pain if tolerated; begin simple, gentle stretches to back. Sit in a chair and move head through the different ranges of motion. This includes the chin down to the chest, extending the head backward, tilting the head side-to-side and rotating the head to each side. Perform 10 repetitions and/or hold each movement for a count of 10 and repeat twice each day. **4. Calcium / magnesium combo:** 3-4 softgels/caps each day with food in divided doses. Get at least 750-1000 mg of calcium and 400-500 mg of magnesium. **5. Massage Therapy:** 1/2 to full hour therapeutic massage to the both the effected area and the body as a whole.
Radicular / Referred Pain	**1. Ice:** Apply a pliable ice pack to the effected area. Place a paper towel or thin cloth between the skin and the ice pack. Ice for 20 minutes at a time. Can repeat 20 minutes every hour or every other hour in first 24 hours. **2. Chiropractic:** Have the effected area evaluated and adjusted by a chiropractor. Follow any instructions they may give in regard to the adjustment and adjunct care. **3. White willow bark:** Take 1-2 caps 3 times /day in first 24 hours. *Caution: If you have a history of ulcers or other gastrointestinal disorder which precludes you from taking aspirin, do not use.* **4. Bromelain:** Take 2 caps 3 times /day in first 24 hours. **5. Herbal Combination:** Valerian,	**1. Chiropractic:** Continue chiropractic adjustments. May need 2-3 per week for period of time. **2. Topically:** Apply arnica montana cream over effected area. Repeat 4-5 times within initial 24 hours. Alternative: Apply wintergreen oil or peppermint oil over effected area with same dosage. **3. Stretching:** Begin on day 3 after beginning of pain if tolerated; begin simple, gentle stretches to back. Perform 10 repetitions and/or hold each movement for a count of 10 and repeat twice each day. **4. Calcium / Magnesium Combo:** Take 3-4 softgels/caps daily with food in divided doses. Get at least 750-1000 mg calcium and 400-500 mg magnesium. **5. Homeopathy:** Take Nerve Tonic 6c to 12c. Take 3-4 tables under tongue 4

COMPLAINT	IMMEDIATE RELIEF	SECONDARY RELIEF
Radicular/ Referred Pain Cont.	hops and skullcap: 2 caps 3 times/day in first 24 hours. Alternative: Drink herbal tea (equal parts chamomile, lemon balm and passionflower) steeped in 6-8 ozs of water for 10 minutes, drink 3 cups /day.	times /day.
Sciatica	**1. Ice:** Apply a pliable ice pack to the effected area. Place a paper towel or thin cloth between the skin and the ice pack. Ice for 20 minutes at a time. Can repeat 20 minutes every hour or every other hour in first 24 hours. **2. Chiropractic:** Have the effected area evaluated and adjusted by a chiropractor. Follow any instructions they may give in regard to the adjustment and adjunct care. **3. Bromelain:** Take 2 caps 3 times /day in first 24 hours. **5. Herbal Combination:** Valerian, hops and skullcap: 2 caps 3 times/day in first 24 hours. Alternative: Drink herbal tea (equal parts chamomile, lemon balm and passionflower) steeped in 6-8 ozs of water for 10 minutes, drink 3 cups /day.	**1. Chiropractic:** Continue chiropractic adjustments. May need 2-3 per week for period of time. **2. DLPA:** Take one cap 375 mg 2 times /day. **3. Stretching:** Begin on day 3 after beginning of pain if tolerated; begin simple, gentle stretches to back. Perform the low back stretches and movements. Do 10 repetitions and/or hold each movement for a count of 10 and repeat twice each day. **4. Calcium / magnesium combo:** Take 3-4 softgels/caps daily with food in divided doses. Get at least 750-1000 mg of calcium and 400-500 mg of magnesium. **5. Homeopathy:** Take Nerve Tonic 6c to 12c. Take 3-4 tables under tongue (sublingual) 4 times cap/day.

CHEST, CIRCULATORY & RESPIRATORY SYSTEMS

Angina	**1. Immediately Rest** by sitting down or lying down. *This may be an emergency situation. Contact your doctor immediately.*	**1. Coenzyme Q10:** Take one cap 100 mg, 1-2 times cap/day. **2. Garlic:** Take one cap 3 times /day. **3. Hawthorn:** Take 1 cap 3 times/day. **4. Calcium / Magnesium Combo:** Take 3 /day. Make sure that the calcium level is 1000 mg and the magnesium is 400-500 mg. **5. Lecithin/Choline/Inositol:** Take these in combination 3 a day.
Bronchitis, Coughing, and Pain	**1. White willow bark** and boneset herb for pain. 1-2 caps of each, 3 times/day. **2. Poultice:** Use the following herbs placed over the chest: 1 part each of lobelia, marshmallow root, slippery elm and burdock. Place herbs in cotton gauze or cheesecloth mesh, soak with hot water, place over chest as it cools, place plastic wrap over this, then a heating pad. Leave on 30 minutes. **3. Herbals Internally:** Make a combination of the following using the following: 2 ozs of licorice; and 1 oz of	**1.** Drink plenty of fluids. **2.** Get plenty of rest. **3.** Utilize postural drainage positions. This is dangling your upper body over the edge of the bed toward the floor with a container to catch the mucus drainage. **4. Vitamin C:** Take one 500 mg cap every 2-3 hours; up to 4000-5000 mg/day. **5. Zinc Lozenges:** Take 1 lozenge every two hours. Zinc content must be at least 20-25 mg of elemental zinc.

135

COMPLAINT	IMMEDIATE RELIEF	SECONDARY RELIEF
Bronchitis Coughing, and Pain Cont.	each of the following: wild cherry bark, slippery elm, horehound, lobelia and coltsfoot. Mix and boil in 3-4 cups of water for 3 minutes, then steep for 10 minutes. Drink 1 cup every 2-3 hours. **4. Bromelain:** 2 caps 2 times /day. **5. Homeopathy:** Take Bryonia alba at 12c up to 30c; under the tongue, 3-4 pellets 4 times/day.	
Myocardial Infarction (Heart Attack)	*This is a medical emergency. Contact 911 and immediately seek medical attention.*	**1. Magnesium:** 500 mg 2 times /day. Can also be used in emergency treatment procedures. **2. Omega 3 Fatty Acids:** 1,000 mg.l 3 times /day. **3. Vitamin B6, B12 and Folic Acid:** 1100 mg of vitamin B6; 1 cap which combines vitamin B12 (2,000-5,000 mcg), folic acid (800 mcg) /day. **4. Ginkgo Biloba:** 1 60 mg, cap extract, 3 times /day. **5. Co Q10:** 100 mg, 1-2 times /day.

HEAD & RELATED STRUCTURES (EARS, EYES, FACE, JAW, MOUTH, NOSE & SINUSES)

COMPLAINT	IMMEDIATE RELIEF	SECONDARY RELIEF
Headache	**1. Feverfew:** 2 caps 3 times /day in first 24 hours. Alternative: In tincture form, 1 dropper full 3-4 times /day. **2. Lavender:** Place 3-4 drops lavender oil on each temple and frontal area of head. Repeat every 2-3 hours. **3. Chiropractic:** Have the effected area evaluated and adjusted by a chiropractor, especially the cervical region. **4. Ginkgo Biloba:** 60 mg, extract, 2-3 times within first 24 hours. **5. Homeopathic:** Belledonna: 12c up to 30c; 3-4 pellets every 1-2 hours for first 6 hours, then same dosage every 2-4 hours during first day.	**1. Omega 3 Fatty Acids:** Take one softgel 3 times /day. **2. Coenzyme Q10:** Take one cap 60-100 mg 1 time /day. **3. DMG (Dimethylglycine):** Take one cap 125 mg 2 times /day. **4. Lecithin/Choline/Inositol:** Take 3-6 softgels /day. **5. Vitamin B3:** Take niacin, one cap 100 mg 1 time /day.
Sinus Headache	**1. Lavender/Wintergreen/Peppermint:** Apply oil across the sinus regions 3-4 times /day. **2. Homeopathic:** Kali bichromicum: 12c to 30c, 3-4 pellets under the tongue (sublingual) every 2-3 hours within the first 24 hours. **3. Homeopathic:** Take cell salt Nat Sulph:3-4 tabs under the tongue (sublingual) 3-4 times /day. **4. Steam Inhaler:** Use a steam inhaler machine and add in wintergreen oil. Sit with machine for 10-20	**1. Vitamin A:** Take 1-2 caps, up to 25,000 IU, 1 time /day. **2. Vitamin C:** Take one 500 mg cap every 2-3 hours; up to 4000-5000 mg/day. **3. Herbal Immune Combo:** Echinacea, goldenseal, astragalus and schizandra: 2-3 caps, 3 times /day. **4. Cayenne:** Take 1 cap 40,000 heat units, 3 times /day. **5. Massage Therapy:** Utilize self-massage by applying pressure to th sinuses and surrounding areas of the head. Do

COMPLAINT	IMMEDIATE RELIEF	SECONDARY RELIEF
Sinus Headache Cont.	minute periods 4-6 times /day in first 24 hours. **5. Moist Heat:** Apply moist heat pad across involved sinuses for 10 minutes at a time, 3-5 times or as needed during the first 24 hours.	this in 3 minute increments and repeat as needed.
Tension Headache	**1. White willow bark/Feverfew:** 1-2 caps of each herb, 3 times /day. *See previous precautions in regard to white willow bark usage.* **2. Homeopathic:** Gelsemium 6c up to 30c; 3-4 pellets/tables under the tongue (sublingual) every 2-3 hours in the first 24 hours. Also cell salt Mag Phos (magnesium phosphate); 3-4 tabs under the tongue (sublingual) every 2-3 hours in the first 24 hours. **3. Ice:** Apply a pliable ice pack to the effected area. Place a paper towel or thin cloth between the skin and the ice pack. Ice for 20 minutes at a time. Can repeat 20 minutes every hour or every other hour in first 24 hours. **4. Lavender/Wintergreen/Peppermint:** Apply oil across the back of neck and base of neck 3-4 times /day. **5. Chiropractic:** Have the effected area evaluated and adjusted by a chiropractor. Follow any instructions they may give in regard to the adjustment and adjunct care.	**1. Chiropractic:** Continue chiropractic adjustments. May need 2-3 per week for period of time. **2. Topically:** Apply arnica montana cream over effected area. Repeat 4-6 times cap/day as needed. **3. Stretching:** Begin on day 3 after beginning of pain if tolerated; begin simple, gentle stretches to back. Sit in a chair and move head through the different ranges of motion. This includes the chin down to the chest, extending the head backward, tilting the head side-to-side and rotating the head to each side. Perform 10 repetitions and/or hold each movement for a count of 10 and repeat twice each day. **4. Calcium / Magnesium Combo:** 3-4 softgels/caps each day with food in divided doses. Get at least 1000 mg of calcium and 400-500 mg of magnesium. **5. Massage Therapy:** 1/2 to 1 hour therapeutic massage to the both the effected area and the body as a whole.
EARS **Middle Ear Infection**	**1. Herbal:** Use garlic/mullein ear oil: place 1-2 drops in both ears 2-3 times /day. Make sure the last application is at bedtime. Use cotton balls, loosely in ear canals to keep oil in the ears. **2 Heat:** Use a heating pad for 10-30 minutes over the effected ear. Place a towel over the heating pad and between it and the effected ear. **3 Homeopathic:** Aconite 12c up to 30c, belladonna 12c up to 30c and pulsatilla 6c up to 12 c; 3-4 pellets of each under the tongue (sublingual) every 3-4 hours during the first 24 hours.	**1. Vitamin A:** Take up to 50,000 IU, one time /day. *Use caution with taking a high dose of vitamin A; especially with children.* **2. Vitamin C:** 500 mg every 2-3 hours; up to 4,000-5,000 mg /day. **3. Herbal Immune Combination:** Take 2-3 caps, 3 times /day of the following: Echinacea, goldenseal, astragalus and schizandra. **4. Zinc:** 30-40 mg /day. **5. Thymus Extract:** 300-500 mg /day.
Swimmer's Ear	**1. Herbal:** Use garlic/mullein ear oil: See above. **2. Heat:** Use a heating pad for 10-30 minutes over the effected ear. Place a towel over the heating pad and	**1. Vitamin A:** Take up to 50,000 IU, one time /day. *Use caution with taking a high dose of vitamin A; especially with children.* **2. Vitamin C:** 500 mg cap every 2-3

COMPLAINT	IMMEDIATE RELIEF	SECONDARY RELIEF
Swimmer's Ear Cont.	between it and the effected ear. **3. Homeopathic:** Aconite 12c up to 30c, belledonna 12c up to 30c and pulsatilla 6c up to 12 c; 3-4 pellets of each under the tongue (sublingual) every 3-4 hours during the first 24 hours.	hours; up to 4,000-5,000 mg /day. **3. Herbal Immune Combination:** Take 2-3 caps, 3 times /day of the following h: Echinacea, goldenseal, astragalus and schizandra. **4. Zinc:** 30-40 mg /day. **5. Thymus Extract:** 300-500 mg /day.
EYES **Conjunctivitis**	**1. Herbal:** Create am herbal liquid eye wash:2 parts eyebright, 1 part of goldenseal, boil in 6-8 ozs of water for 2-3 minutes, then steep for 10 minutes. Let cool. Use an "eye glass" and flush the eye for approximately 30 seconds; repeat twice. Alternative: 1 tbs goldenseal, one teas. salt and 250 mg of vitamin C in 1 quart of water. Let settle. Wash eye out several times /day (from Joseph Pizzorno, N.D.). **2. Heat:** Apply dry heat pad with towel cover over the effected eye for 10 minutes; repeat 2-3 times /day. **3. Topical:** Peel and grate a fresh cucumber; place grated cucumber in large sterile gauze pad or boiled cheesecloth. Squeeze a few drops of cucumber juice directly into the eye. Repeat 2-3 times daily. Alternative: Use same procedure with an organic white potato.	**1. Zinc:** 30-40 mg 1 time /day. **2. Vitamin A:** Take 1-2 caps, up to 50,000 IU (+), 1 time/day. *Use caution with taking a high dose of vitamin A; especially with children. If using above 50,000 IU /day, only take under the direction of a health care professional.* **3. Bilberry:** Take 1 cap, extracted form, 60 mg 1 time /day. **4. Acupuncture:** Utilize acupuncture treatments for overall eye health. Use only a qualified practitioner of Acupuncture. Multiple visits may be required. **5. Vitamin C:** 500 mg every 2-3 hours; up to 4,000-5,000 mg /day.
Eye Injuries	**1. Herbal:** Create a liquid eye wash: (See above) **2. Heat:** Apply dry heat pad with towel cover over the effected eye for 10 minutes; repeat 2-3 times /day. **3. Topical:** See Above	**1. Homeopathic:** Take Aconite 6c up to 12c; 3-4 pellets/tabs under the tongue (sublingual) 3-4 times /day. **2. Zinc:** Take 30-40 mg 1 time /day. **3. Vitamin A:** Take up to 50,000 IU, 1 time /day. *Use caution with taking a high dose of vitamin A; especially with children. Use above 50,000 IU /day only under the direction of a health care professional.* **4. Bilberry:** 60 mg extract, 1 time /day. **5. Vitamin C** 500 mg every 2-3 hours; up to 4,000-5,000 mg /day.
Eye Strain and Pain	**1. Herbal:** Create a liquid eye wash (see above). **2. Heat:** Apply dry heat pad with towel cover over the effected eye for 10 minutes; repeat 2-3 times /day. **3. Topical:** See above	**1. Homeopathic:** Take Ruta graveolens, arnica and apis mellifica, 6c up to 12c; 3-4 pellets/tabs 3-4 times /day. **2. Zinc:** 30-40 mg 1 time /day. **3. Vitamin A:** Take up to 50,000 IU, 1 time /day. *Use caution... see above* **4. Bilberry:** 60 mg extract 1 time /day. **5. Vitamin C:** 500 mg every 2-3

COMPLAINT	IMMEDIATE RELIEF	SECONDARY RELIEF

FACE AND JAW

Temporal-Mandibular Joint Pain & Dysfunction (TMJ)

IMMEDIATE RELIEF:

1. Ice: Use a water frozen in a cup, then peeled to expose a layer of the ice. Apply the ice directly over the effected TMJ joint(s) in revolving, continuous movement. Apply for 3-5 minutes 4-6 times /day. Use in conjunction with heat. Begin with ice -finish with ice (contrast therapy).

2. Heat: Apply a moist heat pack, with a towel covering it, directly over the effected TMJ joint(s) for 10-15 minutes, 3-4 times /day. Use in conjunction with ice.

3. DLPA: 375 mg 1-2 times /day.

4. Wintergreen/Peppermint: Apply 3-5 drops either wintergreen or peppermint oil directly over the effected TMJ joint(s), 4-8 times/day.

5. Herbal Combination: Take a Valerian, hops and skullcap: 2 caps 3 times /day in first 24 hours. Alternative: Drink tea with lemon balm, chamomile, and passion-flower; 1 part of each steeped in 6-8 ozs of water for 10 min, drink 3 cups /day.

SECONDARY RELIEF:

hours; up to 4,000-5,000 mg/day.

1. Calcium / Magnesium Combo: 3-4 softgels/caps each day with food in divided doses. Get at least 1000 mg of calcium and 400-500 mg of magnesium.

2. Vitamin B-Complex: 100 mg /day.

3. Glucosamine/Chondroitin Sulfate: Take in combination 2-3 caps /day. 1,500-2,000 mg of glucosamine sulfate and 1,000-1,500 mg of chondroitin sulfate.

4. Omega 3 Fatty Acids: Take 1,000 mg. 3 times /day.

5. Decrease stress levels; do not chew gum or eat sunflower seeds that need to be deshelled; stop grinding and teeth clenching, etc.

Trigeminal Neuritis and Neuralgia

IMMEDIATE RELIEF:

1. DLPA: 375 mg 1-2 times /day.

2. Wintergreen/Peppermint: Apply 3-5 drops of either wintergreen or peppermint oil directly over the effected TMJ joint(s), 4-8 times /day.

3. Herbal Combination: Valerian, hops and skullcap: 2 caps 3 times /day in first 24 hours. Alternative: Drink herbal tea combination of chamomile, lemon balm and passionflower; 1 part of each steeped in 6-8 ozs of water for 10 minutes, drink 3 cups /day.

SECONDARY RELIEF:

1. Omega 3 Fatty Acids: 1,000 mg. 3 times /day.

2. CoQ10: 60-100 mg 1 time/day.

3. Vitamin B3: 100 mg 1 time /day.

4. Homeopathic: Take nerve tonic 12c up to 30c, 3-4 pellets/tabs 3-4 times cap/day; and cell salts silica and mag phos (magnesium phosphate), 3-4 tabs 4 times /day.

MOUTH
Cold Sores

IMMEDIATE RELIEF:

1. Topical: Apply 1-3 drops of Tea tree oil directly on cold sore, 4-6 times /day.

2. Topical: Apply L-lysine (amino acid) cream directly on the cold sore, 4-6 times /day.

3. Topical: Apply Colloidal silver directly on the cold sore, 3 times /day.

SECONDARY RELIEF:

1. L-Lysine: 500-1000 mg 2 times/day.

2. Zinc: 30-40 mg /day.

3. Vitamin C: 500 mg every 2-3 hours; up to 4,000-5,000 mg/day.

4. Vitamin B-Complex: 100 mg /day.

5. Herbal Immune Combination: Take 2-3 caps, 3 times /day of the following combination: Echinacea, goldenseal, astragalus and schizandra.

COMPLAINT	IMMEDIATE RELIEF	SECONDARY RELIEF
Pharyngitis Sore Throat Pain	**1. Topical:** Gargle 3-5 times /day with a combination of hot water, one teaspoon of salt and apple cider vinegar. Alternative: Gargle 3-5 times /day with a combination of hot water, with one teaspoon of honey and lemon juice. **2. Zinc Lozenge:** Slowly dissolve 1-2 zinc lozenges in the mouth; 3-4 times /day in the first 24 hours. **3. Topical:** Gargle with licorice, cloves and lavender mixture; 3 times /day. **4. Heat:** Apply heating pad or hot compress directly over throat 3 times /day.	**1. Herbal Immune Combination:** Take 2-3 caps, 3 times /day of the following combination: Echinacea, goldenseal, astragalus and schizandra. **2. Vitamin C:** 500 mg cap every 2-3 hours; up to 4,000-5,000 mg /day. **3. Vitamin A:** Take up to 50,000 IU, one time /day. *Use caution with taking a high dose of vitamin A; especially with children. If using above 50,000 IU /day, only take under the direction of a health care professional.* **4. Bee Propolis:** Take as directed on label. **5. Garlic:** 2 caps 3 times /day.
Toothache	**1. Topical:** Apply 1-2 drops of clove oil directly on the involved tooth and the gum around the tooth; 3-5 times /day. **2. Poultice**: Create a small herbal poultice with echinacea, goldenseal and mullein herbs. Use 5 drops of each from an alcohol free extract of echinacea and goldenseal and one part bulk mullein and apply to a small gauze, place gauze directly on/over involved tooth. Leave in for 1-2 hours, repeat as needed. **2.** See your dentist if pain persists.	**1. Vitamin A:** Take up to 50,000 IU, one time /day. *Use caution with taking a high dose of vitamin A; especially with children. If using above 50,000 IU /day, only take. under the direction of a health care professional.* **2. Vitamin C:** 500 mg every 2-3 hours; up to 4,000-5,000 mg /day. **3. Vitamin B-Complex:** 100 mg /day. **4. Herbal Immune Combination:** Take 2-3 caps, 3 times /day of the following h: Echinacea, goldenseal, astragalus and schizandra. **5. Zinc:** Take 1 cap 30 mg /day. **6.** See your dentist and hygienist on a regular basis.

NOSE AND SINUS

COMPLAINT	IMMEDIATE RELIEF	SECONDARY RELIEF
Nose Trauma and Pain	**1. Ice:** Apply a pliable ice pack to the effected area. Place a paper towel or thin cloth between the skin and the ice pack. Ice for 10 minutes at a time. Can repeat 10 minutes every hour or every other hour in first 24 hours. **2. White willow bark:** Take 1-2 caps 3 times /day in first 24 hours. Caution: If you have a history of ulcers or other gastrointestinal disorder which precludes you from taking aspirin, do not use. **3. Bromelain:** Take 2 caps 3 times /day in first 24 hours. **4. Poultice:** Create an herbal poultice using mullein, slippery elm, burdock root and marshmallow. Use one part of each herb, place in a cotton gauze or cheesecloth; apply hot water, let cool; then	**1. Calcium / Magnesium Combo**: Take 3-4 softgels/caps each day with food in divided doses. Get at least 750-1000 mg of calcium and 400-500 mg of magnesium. **2. Lavender:** Place lavender oil, approximately 3-4 drops on the nose. Repeat every 2-3 hours. **3. Vitamin C:** 500 mg every 2-3 hours; up to 4,000-5,000 mg /day. **4. Homeopathic:** Take arnica and ledum 30c each; 3-4 pellets under the tongue (sublingual) 3-4 times /day. **5. Vitamin B-Complex:** 100 mg /day.

COMPLAINT	IMMEDIATE RELIEF	SECONDARY RELIEF
Nose Trauma and Pain Cont.	apply directly over effected area. **5. Homeopathic:** Apply arnica oil/cream directly over the nose and surrounding tissue; 3 times /day.	
Sinusitis and Sinus Pain	**1. Lavender/Wintergreen/Pepper-mint:** Apply oil across the sinus regions 3-4 times /day. **2. Homeopathic:** Kali bichromicum (potassium bichromate) 12c to 30c, 3-4 pellets under the tongue every 2-3 hours within the first 24 hours. **3. Homeopathic:** Cell salt-Nat Sulph (sodium sulfate): 3-4 tabs under the tongue 3-4 times /day. **4. Steam Inhaler:** Add wintergreen oil to a steam inhaler machine. Sit with machine for 10-20 minutes 4-6 times /day in first 24 hours. **5. Moist Heat:** Apply moist heat pad across involved sinuses for 10 minutes at a time, 3-5 times or as needed during the first 24 hours.	**1. Vitamin A:** Take up to 25,000 IU, 1 time /day. **2. Vitamin C:** 500 mg every 2-3 hours; up to 4,000-5,000 mg /day. **3. Herbal Immune Combination:** Take 2-3 caps, 3 times /day of the following herbs: Echinacea, goldenseal, astragalus and schizandra. **4. Cayenne:** 40,000 heat units, 3 times /day. **5. Massage Therapy:** Utilize self-massage by applying pressure to th sinuses and surrounding areas of the head. Do this in 3 minute increments and repeat as needed.

JOINTS & BONES

Osteoarthritis	**1. Heat:** Apply dry or moist heat pad directly over the effected areas. Place a towel between skin and heating pad; 3-5 times /day. **2. Topical:** Apply 5-10 drops of either wintergreen or peppermint oil directly onto the effected areas 3-4 times /day. **3. Topical:** Apply capsicum ointment directly over the effected areas; apply liberally; 3-4 times /day. **4. Homeopathic:** Apply arnica montana gel/cream directly to the effected areas, apply liberally; 3-4 times /day.	**1. Calcium / Magnesium combo:** Take at least 1,000 mg of calcium and 400-500 mg of magnesium, 3-4 soft-gels/caps each day with food in divided doses. **2. Glucosamine/Chondroitin Sulfate:** Take in combination 2-3 caps /day. Take at least 1,500-2,000 mg of glucosamine sulfate and 1,000-1,500 mg of chondroitin sulfate. **3. Omega 3 Fatty Acids:** 1,000 3 times /day. **4. MSM:** 500 -1,000 mg 2 times /day. **5. DLPA:** 375 mg 2 times /day.
Bone and Joint Injuries	**1. Ice:** Apply a pliable ice pack to the effected area. Place a paper towel or thin cloth between the skin and the ice pack. Ice for 10 minutes at a time. Can repeat 10 minutes every hour or every other hour in first 24 hours. **2. White willow bark:** Take 1-2 caps 3 times /day in first 24 hours. *Caution: If you have a history of ulcers or other gastrointestinal disorder which precludes you from taking aspirin, do not use.* **3. Bromelain:** Take 2 caps 3 times /day in first 24 hours. **4. Poultice:** Create an herbal poultice	**1. Calcium / Magnesium Combo:** Take at least 1000 mg of calcium and 400-500 mg of magnesium, 3-4 soft-gels/caps each day with food in divided doses. **2.Glucosamine/Chondroitin Sulfate:** Take in combination 2-3 caps /day. Need to get at least 1,500-2,000 mg of glucosamine sulfate and ,1000-1,500 mg of chondroitin sulfate. **3. Omega 3 Fatty Acids:** 1,000mg 3 times /day. **4. MSM:** 500-1,000 mg 2 times /day. **5. Homeopathic:** Calc fluor (calcium fluoride) 3-4 times /day.

COMPLAINT	IMMEDIATE RELIEF	SECONDARY RELIEF
Bone and Joint Injuries Cont.	using boneset, mullein, slippery elm, burdock root and thyme; use 1 part of each herb, place in a cotton gauze or cheesecloth; apply hot water, let cool; then apply directly. **5. Homeopathic:** Apply arnica oil/cream directly over the nose and surrounding tissue; 3 times /day.	
Gout	**1. Topical:** Create and apply a paste by mixing cayenne (capsicum) powder with 10-20 drops of wintergreen oil; apply directly onto the effected areas 3-4 times /day. *May initially cause stinging which should diminish with use.* **2. Poultice:** Create an herbal poultice using boneset, mullein, slippery elm, burdock root and thyme; use one part of each herb, place in a cotton gauze or cheesecloth; apply hot water, let cool; then apply directly over effected area. **3. Homeopathic:** Apply arnica oil/cream directly over the nose and surrounding tissue; 3 times /day. **4. Bromelain:** Take 2 caps 3 times /day in first 24 hours. **5. Ice:** Apply a pliable ice pack to the effected area. Place a thin cloth between the skin and the ice pack. Ice for 20 minutes at a time. Can repeat ice procedure 4-6 times /day.	**1. Alfalfa:** 400-500 mg; 2 times /day. **2. Omega 3 Fatty Acids:** 1,000 mg. 3 times /day. **3. MSM:** 500-1,000 mg. 2 times /day. **4. Vitamin B-Complex:** 100 mg 1 time /day. **5. Homeopathy:** Take belladonna, nux vomica, calcarea fluorica and colchicum, all from 6c up to 12 c; 3-4 times /day.
Rheumatoid Arthritis	**1. Topical:** Create and apply a paste by mixing cayenne (capsicum) powder with 10-20 drops of wintergreen oil; apply directly onto the effected areas 3-4 times /day. *May initially cause stinging which should diminish with use.* **2. Poultice:** Create an herbal poultice using boneset, mullein, slippery elm, burdock root and thyme; use 1 part of each, place in a cotton gauze or cheesecloth; apply hot water, let cool; then apply directly. **3. Homeopathy:** Apply arnica oil/cream directly over the nose and surrounding tissue; 3 times /day. **4. Bromelain:** Take 2 caps 3 times /day in first 24 hours. **5. Ice:** Apply a pliable ice pack to the effected area. Place a paper towel or thin cloth between the skin and the ice pack. Ice for 20 min. Can repeat ice procedure 4-6 times /day.	**1. Alfalfa:** Take two caps 400-500 mg each; 2 times /day. **2. Omega 3 Fatty Acids:** 1,000 mg 3 times /day. **3. MSM:** 500-1,000 mg 2 times /day. **4. Vitamin B-Complex:** 100 mg 1 time /day. **5. Homeopathy:** Take belladonna, nux vomica, calcarea fluorica and colchicum, all from 6c up to 12 c; 3-4 times /day.

COMPLAINT	IMMEDIATE RELIEF	SECONDARY RELIEF

LOWER EXTREMITIES: HIPS, THIGHS, KNEES, CALVES, ANKLES, FEET & TOES

COMPLAINT	IMMEDIATE RELIEF	SECONDARY RELIEF
Ankle Sprain	**1. Ice:** Apply a pliable ice pack to the effected area. Place a paper towel or thin cloth between the skin and the ice pack. Ice for 20 minutes at a time. Can repeat 20 minutes every hour or every other hour in first 24 hours. **2. Wrap** effected area in an ace bandage firmly to apply compression and keep elevated. **3. White willow bark:** Take 1-2 caps 3 times /day in first 24 hours. *Caution: If you have a history of ulcers or other gastrointestinal disorder which precludes you from taking aspirin, do not use.* **4. Bromelain:** Take 2 caps 3 times /day in first 24 hours. **5. Topically:** Apply arnica montana cream over effected area. Repeat 4-5 times within initial 24 hours.	**1. B-complex:** 50-100 mg /day. **2. Vitamin C:** Use a calcium or potassium ascorbate form (buffered). Take up to bowel tolerance. If you are currently not taking vitamin C, begin with one 500 mg cap /day; up to 3000-5000 mg /day. **3. Stretching:** Begin stretching/flexibility movements by day 2 or 3, depending on tolerance. Use abbreviated, gentle motions. Perform 10 repetitions and/or hold each movement for a count of 10 and repeat twice. Slowly increase amount of motion over time. **4. MSM:** 500-1,000 mg 2 times /day. **5. Exercise:** Begin gentle exercise program to effected area soft tissue. Depending on area impacted, this will involve some type of progressive, resistance training.
Foot and Heel Pain	**1. Ice:** Apply a pliable ice pack to the effected area. Place a paper towel or thin cloth between the Skin and the ice pack. Ice for 20 minutes at a time. Can repeat 20 minutes every hour or every other hour in first 24 hours. **2. Wrap** effected area in an ace bandage firmly to apply compression and keep elevated. **3. White willow bark:** Take 1-2 caps 3 times /day in first 24 hours. *Caution: see above* **4. Bromelain:** Take 2 caps 3 times /day in first 24 hours. **5. Topically:** Apply arnica montana cream over effected area. Repeat 4-5 times within initial 24 hours.	**1. B-complex:** 50-100 mg /day. **2. Vitamin C:** Use a calcium or potassium ascorbate form (buffered). Take up to bowel tolerance. If you are currently not taking vitamin C, begin with one 500 mg cap /day; up to 3,000-5,000 mg /day. **3. Omega 3 Fatty Acids:** 1,000 mg. 3 times /day. **4. MSM:** 500-1,000 mg 2 times /day. **5. Homeopathic:** Calc fluor (calcium fluoride) 3-4 times /day.
Hip Pain	**1. Ice:** Apply a pliable ice pack to the effected area. Place a paper towel or thin cloth between the skin and the ice pack. Ice for 20 minutes at a time. Can repeat 20 minutes every hour or every other hour in first 24 hours. **2. Chiropractic:** Have the effected area evaluated and adjusted by a chiropractor. Follow any instructions they may give in regard to the adjustment and adjunct care. **3. White willow bark:** Take 1-2 caps 3 times /day in first 24 hours.	**1. Chiropractic:** Continue chiropractic adjustments. May need 2-3 per week for period of time. **2. Topically:** Apply arnica montana cream over effected area. Repeat 4-5 times within initial 24 hours. Alternative: Apply wintergreen oil or peppermint oil over effected area with same dosage. **3. Stretching:** Begin on day 3 after beginning of pain if tolerated; begin simple, gentle stretches to the hip region. Lie on your back on the bed. Bring each knee to the chest and hold;

COMPLAINT	IMMEDIATE RELIEF	SECONDARY RELIEF
Hip Pain Cont.	*Caution: If you have a history of ulcers or other gastrointestinal disorder which precludes you from taking aspirin, do not use.* **4. Bromelain:** Take 2 caps 3 times /day in first 24 hours. **5. Herbal Combination:** Combine valerian, hops and skullcap: Take 2 caps 3 times /day in first 24 hours. Alternative: Drink herbal tea combination of chamomile, lemon balm and passionflower; one part of each steeped in 6-8 ozs of water for 10 minutes, drink 3 cups /day.	bring both knees to the chest and hold; place the bottom of your feet together and bend your knees in a frog-leg position; lie on the edge of the bed and let one leg at a time stretch over the side, etc. Perform 10 repetitions and/or hold each movement for a count of 10 and repeat twice each day. **4. Calcium / Magnesium Combo:** Take 3-4 softgels/caps each day with food in divided doses. Get at least 750-1000 mg of calcium and 400-500 mg of magnesium. **5. Massage Therapy:** 1/2 to 1 hour therapeutic massage to the both the effected area and the body as a whole.
Intermittent Claudication	**1. Stop walking movement;** sit or lie down and rest for a period of 5-10 minutes.	**1. Ginkgo Biloba:** Take one cap 60 mg, extracted form, 2-3 times /day. **2. Vitamin C:** Use a calcium or potassium ascorbate form (buffered). Take up to bowel tolerance. If you are currently not taking vitamin C, begin with one 500 mg /day; up to 3,000 to 5,000 mg /day. **3. Omega 3 Fatty Acids:** 1,000 mg 3 times /day. **4. CoQ10:** 100 mg, 1-2 times /day. **5. Garlic:** Take 1 cap 3 times /day.
Knee Pain	**1. Ice:** Apply a pliable ice pack to the effected area. Place a paper towel or thin cloth between the skin and the ice pack. Ice for 20 minutes at a time. Can repeat 20 minutes every hour or every other hour in first 24 hours. **2. White willow bark:** 1-2 caps 3 times /day in first 24 hours. *Caution: If you have a history of ulcers or other gastrointestinal disorder which precludes you from taking aspirin, do not use.* **3. Bromelain:** Take 2 caps 3 times /day in first 24 hours. **4. Topically:** Apply arnica montana cream over effected area. Repeat 4-5 times within initial 24 hours. **5. Wrap** knee if needed and keep elevated.	**1. Topically:** Apply peppermint oil or capsicum over effected area 3 times /day. **2. Calcium / Magnesium Combo:** Take at least 750-1000 mg of calcium and 400-500 mg of magnesium.each day with food in divided doses. **3. Omega 3 Fatty Acids:** 1,000 3 times /day. **4. MSM:** 500 mg 2 times /day. **5. Homeopathic:** Calc fluor (calcium fluoride) 3-4 times /day.

COMPLAINT	IMMEDIATE RELIEF	SECONDARY RELIEF

REPRODUCTIVE SYSTEM DISORDERS

COMPLAINT	IMMEDIATE RELIEF	SECONDARY RELIEF
Pregnancy Discomforts	**1. Heat:** Apply dry or moist heat topically to areas of discomfort. Place a towel(s) between heating pad and skin. Apply only for periods of 10 minutes as needed. *Caution: Do not overheat the body.* **2. Ice:** Apply a pliable ice pack to the effected area. Place a paper towel or thin cloth between the skin and the ice pack. Ice for 10 minutes at a time. Repeat as needed. *Caution: Do not over cool the body.* **3. Topically:** Apply arnica montana cream over effected area. Repeat 2-4 times within initial 24 hours. **4. Chiropractic:** Have the effected area, typically the low back, pelvis and mid-back, evaluated and adjusted by a chiropractor. Follow any instructions they may give in regard to the adjustment and adjunct care.	**1. Calcium and Magnesium Combo:** Take at least 500-1,000 mg of calcium and 300-500 mg of magnesium each day with food in divided doses. **2. Omega 3 Fatty Acids:** Take 1,000 mg. 2 times per day. **3. Chiropractic:** Continue chiropractic adjustments. May need 1 or more times per week during the pregnancy. **4. Homeopathic:** Take cell salt mag phos (magnesium phosphate) 2-3 times per day or as directed for pregnancy.
Pre-menstrual Pain and Cramping	**1. Topically:** Apply arnica montana cream over effected area. Repeat 4-5 times within initial 24 hours. Alternative: Apply wintergreen oil or peppermint oil over effected area with same dosage. **2. Omega 3 Fatty Acids:** Take 1,000 mg. 3 times per day. **3. Calcium and Magnesium Combo:** Take at least 1,000 mg of calcium and 500 mg of magnesium each day with food in divided doses. **4. Heat:** Apply moist or day heat to the low back and abdomen/pelvic region. 15-20 minutes at a time 3-4 times per day or as needed. **5. Herbal Combination:** Take a combination of valerian, hops and skullcap: 2 caps 3 times per day in first 24 hours. Alternative: Drink herbal tea combination of chamomile, lemon balm and passionflower; one part of each steeped in 6-8 ounces of water for 10 minutes, drink 3 cups per day.	**1. Chiropractic:** Have the effected area, typically the low back, pelvis and mid-back, evaluated and adjusted by a chiropractor. Follow any instructions they may give in regard to the adjustment and adjunct care. Follow up for continued care as recommended. **2. White willow bark:** Take 1-2 capsules 3 times per day in first 24 hours. Caution: If you have a history of ulcers or other gastrointestinal disorder which precludes you from taking aspirin, do not use. **3. DLPA:** Take one capsule 375 mg 1-2 times per day. **4. Herbal:** Make tea of red raspberry leaves. Take one part (or prepared tea bag) and steep for 5 minutes in 6 ounces of water. Drink 1-2 cups per day. **5. Massage Therapy:** 1/2 to 1 hour therapeutic massage to the both the effected area and the body as a whole.

UPPER EXTREMITIES: SHOULDERS, ARMS, ELBOWS, WRISTS, HAND & FINGERS

COMPLAINT	IMMEDIATE RELIEF	SECONDARY RELIEF
Carpal Tunnel Syndrome	**1. Ice:** Apply a pliable ice pack to the effected area. Place a paper towel or thin cloth between the skin and the ice pack. Ice for 15-20 minutes at a time. Can repeat 20	**1. Ice:** Continue icing each day 3-4 times per day, 15-20 minutes at a time. Place a paper towel or thin cloth between the skin and the ice pack. **2. Ultrasound:** Seek a health care pro-

COMPLAINT	IMMEDIATE RELIEF	SECONDARY RELIEF
Carpal Tunnel Syndrome Cont.	minutes every hour or every other hour in first 24 hours. **2. Bromelain:** Take 2 caps 3 times per day in first 24 hours. **3. Vitamin B6:** 100 mg 2 times during first 24 hours. **4. Brace:** Brace the effected wrist with a "cock-up" splint that has the metal brace within it. **5.** Keep effected limb elevated as much as possible; limit usage to minimal.	fessional (chiropractor or physical therapist) to perform pulsed ultrasound on effect wrist for 3 minute treatments 2-3 times per week. **3. Massage Therapy:** Have massage therapy performed on effected wrist and the upper limb, neck and upper back; 1 hour treatments. **4. Vitamin B6:** 100 mg 1-2 times / day for 4-6 weeks. **5. Stretching:** As swelling and pain decrease, begin gentle, limited range of motion movements on effected wrist. Limit work and usage of effected limb and wrist.
Elbow, Hand & Shoulder Pain	**1. Ice:** Apply a pliable ice pack to the effected area. Place a paper towel or thin cloth between the skin and the ice pack. Ice for 20 minutes at a time. Can repeat 20 minutes every hour or every other hour in first 24 hours. **2. White willow bark:** 1-2 caps 3 times / day in first 24 hours. *Caution: If you have a history of ulcers or other gastrointestinal disorder which precludes you from taking aspirin, do not use.* **3. Bromelain:** Take 2 caps 3 times per day in first 24 hours. **4. Topically:** Apply arnica montana cream over effected area. Repeat 4-5 times within initial 24 hours. **5.** Wrap effected area as needed (hand, wrist and elbow); keep elevated.	**1. Topically:** Apply peppermint oil or capsicum over effected area 3 times /day. **2. Calcium / Magnesium Combo:** Take at least 750-1000 mg of calcium and 400-500 mg of magnesium.each day with food in divided doses. **3. Omega 3 Fatty Acids:** 1,000 3 times / day. **4. MSM:** 1,000 mg. 2 times per day. **5. Glucosamine/Chondroitin Sulfate:** Take in combination 2-3 caps /day. Need to get at least 1,500-2,000 mg of glucosamine sulfate and 1,000-1,500 mg of chondroitin sulfate.

WHOLE BODY

Burns	**1. Clean** burn site and use cool water running over burn for at least 5 minutes or more as needed. **2. Topical:** Apply pure aloe vera gel directly over burn site. Apply liberally 4-6 times during first 24 hours. **3. Topical:** Apply calendula gel/cream directly over burn site. Mix with aloe vera. Apply liberally 4-6 times during first 24 hours. **4. Bromelain:** Take 2 caps 3 times per day in first 24 hours.	**1. Topical:** Apply colloidal silver to burn area. Apply as directed on bottle. **2. Multivitamin and mineral complex.** Take 1-2 softgels/caps / day or as directed on bottle to get adequate dose. Need additional vitamin A (50,000 IU's (+)), beta-carotene (25,000 IU), vitamin C (4000-5000 mg), vitamin E (800-1200 IU) and all the B vitamins (100 mg); all per day. **3. Zinc:** 30 mg 3 times / day until burned region is healed. **4. Amino Acid Complex:** Take a free-form amino acid complex containing all of the essential and non-essential amino acids . **5. Essential Fatty Acids:** 2,000 mg 2 times /day. Use flaxseed or primrose oil.

COMPLAINT	IMMEDIATE RELIEF	SECONDARY RELIEF
Fibromyalgia Syndrome	**1. Ice:** Apply a pliable ice pack to the effected area. Place a paper towel or thin cloth between the skin and the ice pack. Ice for 20 minutes at a time. Can repeat 20 minutes every hour or every other hour in first 24 hours. **2. Bromelain:** Take 2 capsules 3 times per day in first 24 hours. **3. White willow bark:** Take 1-2 capsules 3 times per day in first 24 hours. *Caution: If you have a history of ulcers or other gastrointestinal disorder which precludes you from taking aspirin, do not use.* **4. Heat:** Apply dry or moist heat pad directly over the effected areas. Place a towel between skin and heating pad; 3-5 times per day. **5. DLPA:** 375 mg. 2 times first 24 hours.	**1. Calcium and Magnesium Combo:** Take at least 1,000 mg of calcium and 500 mg of magnesium each day with food in divided doses **2. Omega 3 Fatty Acids:** Take one softgel 3 times per day. **3. MSM:** 1,000 mg. 2 times / day. **4. Malic Acid:** 250 mg. 3 times per day. **5. Chiropractic:** Have the effected area(s) evaluated and adjusted by a chiropractor. Follow any instructions they may give in regard to the adjustment and adjunct care. Follow up for continued care as recommended.
Shingles	**1. Topical:** Apply L-lysine cream plus (also has echinacea, vitamin A, zinc and other natural substances within it) to the effected area of vesicle outbreak. Apply 4 times per day. **2. DLPA:** Take one capsule 375 mg two times per day. **3. Quercetin:** 250 mg. 3-4 times /day. **4. Topical:** Apply zinc cream to the effected area of vesicle outbreak. Apply with L-lysine cream 4 times per day. **5. Homeopathic:** Take arnica montana 30c; 3-4 pellets as directed on the bottle (may be every hour or every two hours for this condition).	**1. Homeopathic:** Take the following at 12c to 30c dosages, 3-4 pellets/tables 4 times per day – Arsenicum album 12c; Apis mellifica 30c; Rhus toxicodendron 12c; and Mezereum 30c. **2. L-Lysine:** Take internally (oral) dose, 500 mg. 2-3 times per day. **3. Herbal Immune Combination:** Take 2-3 caps, 3 times per day of the following herbs in combination – Echinacea, goldenseal, astragalus and schizandra. **4. Herbal Combination:** Take a herbal combination of valerian, hops and skullcap – Take 2 capsules 3 times per day in first 24 hours. Alternative: Drink herbal tea combination of chamomile, lemon balm and passionflower; one part of each steeped in 6-8 ozs. of water for 10 minutes, drink 3 cups per day. **5.** Continue all initial topical measures until vesicles have dried and resolved.

Bibliography

Section I

1. Guyton, A., M.D., "The Nervous System – Chapter 41," in Textbook of Medical Physiology, 6th Ed.; Philadelphia: W.B Saunders Company, 1981.

2. Price, SA., and Wilson, LM., Pathophysiology Clinical Concepts Of Disease Properties, 3rd Ed.; New York: McGraw-Hill Book Company, 1986.

3. McNaught, AB., and Callander, R., Illustrated Physiology, 4th Ed.; New York: Churchill Livingstone, 1983.

4. Cahill, M., et al., Professional Guide To Diseases, 6th ed.; Springhouse, PA: Springhouse Corporation, 1998.

5. Cahill, M., et al., Expert Pain Management, Springhouse, PA: Springhouse Corporation, 1997.

6. Graedon, J., and Graedon, T., The People's Guide To Deadly Drug Interactions, New York: St. Martin's Press, 1995.

7. U.S Pharmacopeia, The USP Guide To Medicines, 1st Ed.; New York: Avon Books, 1996.

8. Rapp, R.P., et al., The Pill Book Guide To Over-The-Counter Medications, 1st Ed.; New York: Bantam Books, 1997.

9. Rybacki, J.J., and Long, J.W., The Essential Guide To Prescription Drugs, 1998 Ed.; New York: HarperCollins Publishers, Inc., 1998.

10. Berkow, R., M.D., et al., The Merck Manual, 15th Ed.; New Jersey: Merck & Co., Inc., 1987.

11. McCullough, K., et al., Dorland's Pocket Medical Dictionary, 23rd Ed.; Philadelphia, PA: W. B. Saunders, Co., 1982.

12. Liska, K., The Pharmacist's Guide To The Most Misused And Abused Drugs In America, New York: Collier Books, Macmillan Publishing Co., 1988.

13. Sharp, B., and Yaksh, T., "Pain killers of the immune system," Nat Med, (8): 831-2, Aug. 3, 1997.

Section II

14. Burton Goldberg Group, et al., Alternative Medicine The Definitive Guide, Fife, WA: Future Medicine Publishing, Inc.,

1994.

15. Murray, M., and Pizzorno, J., Encyclopedia Of Natural Medicine, 2nd Ed.; Rocklin, CA: Prima Publishing, 1998.

16. Atkins, R., M.D., Dr. Atkin's Vita-Nutrient Solution, New York: Simon & Schuster, 1998.

17. Airola, P., How To Get Well, 27th Printing; Sherwood, OR: Health Plus, Publishers, 1996.

18. Null, G., Ultimate Anti-Aging Program, New York: Kensington Publishing Corp., 1999.

19. Barney, P., M.D., Doctor's Guide To Natural Medicine, Pleasant Grove, UT: Woodland Publishing, 1998.

20. Balch, J.F., M.D., and Balch, P.A., Prescription For Nutritional Healing, 2nd Ed.; Garden City Park, New York: Avery Publishing Group, 1997.

21. Christopher, J.R., School Of NaturalHealing, Springville, UT: Christopher Publications, Inc., 1976.

Section III

22. Null, G., The Complete Guide To Health And Nutrition, New York: Dell Publishing, 1984.

23. Mindell, E., Earl Mindell's New And Revised Vitamin Bible, New York: Warner Books, 1985.

24. Balch, J.F., M.D., and Balch, P.A., Prescription For Nutritional Healing A-To-Z Guide To Supplements, Garden Park City, New York: Avery Publishing Group, 1998.

25. Werbach, M.R., M.D., Nutritional Influences On Illness, 2nd Ed.; Tarzana, CA: Third Line Press, 1993.

26. Yanick, J.R., and Jaffe, R., M.D., et al., Clinical Chemistry & Nutrition Guidebook, Vol. 1; T & H Publishing, 1988.

27. Lininger, S., Wright, J., M.D., Brown, D., and Gaby, A., M.D., The Natural Pharmacy, Rocklin, CA: Prima Publishing, 1998.

28. Tenney, L., The Encyclopedia Of Natural Remedies, Pleasant Grove, UT: Woodland Publishing, 1995.

29. Waickman, F.J., M.D., et al., "Nutrition As It Relates To Environmental Medicine – Conference July 25-26, 1990," American Academy Of Environmental Medicine, Denver, CO: Clinical Ecology Publications, Inc., 1990.

30. Lytle, RL., "Chronic dental pain: Possible benefits of food restriction and sodium restriction," J Appl Nutr, 40(2): 95-

98, 1988.

31. Blalock, JE., "Natural painkillers," Nat Med, (12): 1302; Dec. 3, 1997.

32. Creagan, ET., et al., "Failure of high-dose vitamin C (ascorbic acid) therapy to benefit patients with advanced cancer," N Engl J Med, 301: 687-90, 1979.

33. Hanck, A., and Weiser, H., "Analgesic and anti-inflammatory properties of vitamins," Int J Vitam Nutr Res, (suppl) 27: 189-206, 1985.

34. Quirin, H., "Pain and vitamin B1 therapy," Bibl Nutr Dieta (38): 110-1, 1986.

35. Meador, KJ., et al., "Evidence for a central cholinergic effect of high dose thiamine," Ann Neurol, 34, 724-726, 1993.

36. Franchi, G., and Violani, M., "Our clinical experience in the use of high doses of thiamine in anesthesia," Acta Anaesthesiol, (suppl) 1: 67-76, 1968.

37. Bernstein, AL., "Vitamin B6 in neurology," Ann N Y Acad Sci, 585: 250-60, 1990.

38. Ellis, JM., and Folkers, K., "Clinical aspects of treatment of carpal tunnel syndrome with B6," Annuals NY Acad Sci, 585, 302-320, 1990.

39. Jones, CL., and Gonzalez, V., "Pyridoxine deficiency: A new factor in diabetic neuropathy," J Am Pod Assoc, 68, 646-653, 1978.

40. Dettori, AG., and Ponari, O., "Effetto antalgico della cobamamide in corso di neuropatie periferiche di diversa etiopatogenesi," Minerva Med, 64: 1077-82, 1973.

41. Ibid (See number 31)

42. Yaqub, BA., Siddique, A., and Sulimani, R., "Effects of methylcobalamin on diabetic neuropathy," Clin Neurol Neurosurg, 94, 105-111, 1992.

43. Kryzhanovskii, GN., et al., "Endogenous opioid system in the realization of the analgesic effect of alpha-tocopherol," Biull Eksp Biol Med, 105(2): 148-50, 1988.

44. Ayers, S., Jr., and Mihan, R., "Leg cramps (systremma) and restless legs syndrome," California Medicine, Vol. III, No. 2, (August 1969) pp. 87-91.

45. Ibid (See number 31)

46. Chick, LR., and Borah, G., "Calcium carbonate gel therapy for hydrofluoric acid burns of the hand," Plast Reconstr Surg, 86(5): 935-40, Nov. 1990.

47. Abraham, G., "Management of fibromyalgia: Rationale for

the use of magnesium and malic acid," J Nutr Med, 3, 49-59, 1992.

48. Ramadan, NM., et al., "Low brain magnesium in migraine," Headache, 29, 590-593, 1989.

49. Bhathena, S., et al., "Decreased plasma enkephalins in copper deficiency in man," Am J Clin Nutr, 43: 42-46, 1986.

50. Walker, WR., and Keats, DM., "An investigation of the therapeutic value of the copper bracelet – dermal assimilation of copper in arthritic/rheumatoid conditions," Agents and Actions, 6, 454-458, 1976.

51. Jameson, S., et al., "Pain relief and selenium balance in patients with connective tissue disease and osteoarthritis: A double-blind selenium tocopherol supplementation study," Nutr Res, (suppl) 1: 391-97, 1985.

52. Tarp, U., et al., "Selenium treatment in rheumatoid arthritis," Scand J Rheumatol, 14, 364-368, 1985.

53. Hachisu, M., et al., "Analgesic effect of novel organogermanium compound, Ge-132," J Pharmacobiodyn, 6(11): 814-20, 1983.

54. Da Camara, CC., and Dowless, GV., "Glucosamine sulfate for osteoarthritis," Ann Pharmacother, 32(5): 580-7; May 1998.

55. Giordano, N., Nardi, P., Senesi, M., et al., "The efficacy and safety of GS in the treatment of arthritis," Clin Ter, 147: 99-105, 1996.

56. Baici, A., et al., "Analysis of GAGs in human serum after oral administration of chondroitin sulfate," Rheumatology Intl, 12: 81-88, 1992.

57. Conte, A., et al., "Biochemical and pharmacokinetic aspects of oral treatment with chondroitin sulfate," Drug Res, 45: 918-925, 1995.

58. Koesis, JJ., Harkaway, S., and Snyder, R., "Biological effects of the metabolites of dimethylsulfoxide," Ann NY Acad Sci, 1975.

59. Obukowicz, MG., Raz, A., Pyla, PD., Rico, JG., Wendling, JM., and Needleman, P., "Identification and characterization of a novel delta6/delta5 fatty acid desaturase inhibitor as a potential anti-inflammatory agent," Biochem Pharmacol, 55(7): 1045-58, Apr. 1998.

60. Singh, S., and Majumdar, DK., "Evaluation of antiinflammatory activity of fatty acids of ocimum sanctum fixed oil," Indian J Exp Biol, 35(4): 380-3, Apr. 1997.

61. Batmanghelidj, F., How to deal with back pain and rheumatoid joint pain, Falls Church, VA: Global Health Solutions, Inc., 1991.

62. Masson, M., "Bromelain in blunt injuries of the locomotor system – a study of observed applications in general practice," Fortschr Med, 113: 303-306, 1995.

63. Horger, I., "Enzyme therapy in multiple rheumatic diseases," Therapiewoche, 33, 3948-3957, 1983.

64. Budd, K., "Use of D-phenylalanine, an enkephalinase inhibitor, in the treatment of intractable pain," Adv Pain Res Ther, 5: 305-308, 1983.

65. Seltzer, S., et al., "The effects of dietary tryptophan on chronic maxillofacial pain and experimental pain tolerance," J Psychiatr Res, 17: 181-6, 1982-3.

66. De Benedittis, G., and Massei, R., "5-HT precursors in migraine prophylaxis. A double-blind cross-over study with L-5-hydroxytryptphan versus placebo,""Clin J Pain, 3: 123-129, 1986.

67. Hart, O., Mullee, MA., Lewith, G., and Miller, J., "Double-blind, placebo-controlled, randomized clinical trial of homeopathic arnica C30 for pain and infection after total abdominal hysterectomy," J R Soc Med, 90(2): 73-8, Feb. 1997.

68. Sakai, S., "Pharmacological actions of verbena officinalis extracts," Gifu Ika Daigaku Klyo, 11(1): 6-17, 1963.

69. Gupta, I., et al., "Effects of Boswellia serrata gum resin in patients with ulcerative colitis," Eur J Med Res, 2(1): 37-43, Jan. 1997.

70. Felter, HW., The Eclectic Materia Medica, Pharmacology and Therapeutics, Portland, OR: Eclectic Medical Publications, 1983.

71. Fusco, BM., and Giacovazzo, M., "Peppers and pain – The promise of capsicum," Drugs, 53(6): 909-14, June 1997.

72. Forster, HB., et al., "Antispasmodic effects of some medicinal plants," Planta Medica, 40: 309, 1980.

73. Kampf, R., Schweitz Apothek Zeitung, 114: 337, 1976.

74. Murphy, JJ., Hepinstall, S., Mitchell, JR., "Randomized double-blind placebo-controlled trial of feverfew in migraine prevention," Lancet, 23: 189-92, 1988.

75. Chevallier, A., Encyclopedia Of Medicinal Plants, New York, NY: DK Publishing, 1996.

76. Singh, YN., "Effects of kava on neuromuscular transmission and muscle contractility," J Ethnopharmacol, 7(3): 267-

76, 1983.

77. Parmar, SS., Tangri, KK., Seth, PK., and Bhargava, KP., "Biochemical basis for anti-inflammatory effects of glycyrrhetic acid and its derivatives," Int'l Congress Of Bio, 6(5): 410, 1967.

78. Leung, AY., Encyclopedia Of Common Natural Ingredients Used In Food, Drugs And Cosmetics, New York, NY: J. Wiley and Sons, 1980.

79. Hazelhoff, B., et al., "Antispasmodic effects of Valeriana compounts: An in-vivo and in-vitro study on the guinea-pig ileum," Arch Int Pharma, 257: 274, 1982.

80. Schmid, B., and Heide, L., "The use of salicis cortex in rheumatic disease: phytotherapie with know mode of action," PM Abstracts 43rd Ann Congr, 61: 94, 1995.

81. DerMarderosian, A. (Editor), et al., The Review Of Natural Products, St. Louis, MO: Facts and Comparisons Publishing Group, 1998-99.

82. PDR For Herbal Medicines, 1st Ed; Montvale, NJ: Medical Economics Co., 1998.

83. Mowrey, DB., Proven Herbal Blends, New Canaan, CT: Keats Publishing, 1986.

84. Bruning, N., and Weinstein, C., M.D., Healing Homeopathic Remedies, New York, NY: Dell Publishing, 1996.

85. Panos, M., M.D. and Heimlich, J., Homeopathic Medicine At Home, New York: G.P. Putman's Sons, 1980.

86. Weintraub, S., Natural Healing With Cell Salts, Pleasant Grove, UT: Woodland Publishing, Inc., 1996.

87. Plaugher, G., and Lopes, MA., et al., Textbook Of Clinical Chiropractic, Baltimore, Maryland: Williams & Wilkins, 1993.

88. Kisner, C., and Colby, LA., Therapeutic Exercise, 2nd Ed.; Philadelphia, PA: F.A. Davis Co., 1990.

89. Lidell, L., et al., The Book Of Massage – The Complete Step-By-Step Guide To Eastern And Western Techniques, New York, NY: Simon & Schuster, Inc., 1984.

90. Kahn, J., Principles And Practice Of Electrotherapy, New York, NY: Churchill Livingstone, 1987.

RECOMMENDED READING LIST

The following is a list of books that you can utilize for your natural health knowledge and education. There are many other natural health books available beyond what is listed here, so please do not limit yourself to just this list.

General:

Alternative Medicine, The Definitive Guide by The Burton Goldberg Group.

Doctor's Guide To Natural Medicine by Paul Barney, M.D.

Dr. Atkin's Vita-Nutrient Solution by Robert C. Atkins, M.D.

Encyclopedia Of Natural Medicine by Michael Murray, N.D. and Joseph Pizzorno, N.D.

Encyclopedia Of Natural Remedies by Louise Tenney, M.H.

Nutritional Influences On Illness – Second Edition by Melvyn R. Werback, M.D.

Prescription For Natural Healing by James F. Balch, M.D. and Phyliss A. Balch, C.N.C.

School Of Natural Healing, 20th Anniversary Edition by Dr. John R. Christopher.

The Complete Guide To Health And Nutrition By Gary Null.

The Natural Pharmacy by Skye Lininger, D.C., Jonathan Wright, M.D. and Donald Brown, N.D.

Supplements:

A – to – Z Guide To Supplement by James F. Balch, M.D. and Phyllis A. Balch, C.N.C.

Encyclopedia of Nutritional Supplements by Michael Murray, N.D.

Earl Mindell's New and Revised Vitamin Bible by Earl Mindell.

Food And Diet:

Diet and Disease by E. Cheraskin, M.D., D.M.D., W.M. Ringsdorf, Jr., D.M.D. and J.W. Clark, D.D.S.

Diet and Nutrition: A Holistic Approach by Rudolph Ballentine.

Foods That Heal by Dr. Bernard Jensen.

Food and Healing by Annemarie Colbin.

Juices, Teas and Tonics by John Heinerman.

Mastering The Zone by Barry Sears, Ph.D.

Nutrition Almanac, Fourth Edition by Gayla J. Kirschmann and John D. Kirschmann.

Phyto-Nutrients by Beth M. Ley, Ph.D.

Staying Healthy With Nutrition by Elson M. Haas, M.D.

The Complete Raw Juice Therapy by Thorson's Editorial Board.

The Healing Power Of Foods by Michael T. Murray, N.D.

Whole Food Facts, The Complete Reference Guide by Evelyn Roehl.

Your Fat Is Not Your Fault by Carol Simontacchi, C.C.N., M.S.

Herbals:

A Modern Herbal by M. Grieve.

Back to Eden by Jethro Kloss.

Chinese Herbs by John D. Keys.

Chinese Herbal Medicine by Dan Bensky and Andrew Gamble.

Chinese Herbal Remedies by Albert Leung.

Chinese Tonic Herbs by Ron Teeguarden.

Medicinal Plants Of The Mountain West by Michael Moore.

Natural Healing With Herbs by Humbart Santillo, N.D.

Proven Herbal Blends by Daniel B. Mowrey, Ph.D.

The Complete Medicinal Herbal by Penelope Ody.

The Healing Power Of Herbs by Michael T. Murray, N.D.

The Herb Book by John Lust.

The Herbal Medicine Cabinet by Debra St. Claire.

The Holistic Herbal by David Hoffmann.

The Way of Herbs by Michael Tierra, C.A., N.D.

Homeopathic:

Healing Homeopathic Remedies by Nancy Bruning and Corey Weinstein, M.D.

Homeopathic Materia Medica and Repertory by W. Boericke, M.D.

Homeopathic Medicine At Home by Maesimund B. Panos, M.D. and Jane Heimlich.

Homeopathic Remedies For Children's Common Ailments by Carolyn Dean, M.D.

Natural Healing With Cell Salts by Dr. Skye Weintraub.

The Complete Homeopathy Handbook by Miranda Castro.

The Essentials Of Homeopathic Materia Medica by Jacques Jouanny, M.D.

The Family Guide To Homeopathy by Alain Horvilleur, M.D.

Other Books:

Alternative Medicine Guide – Chronic Fatigue, Fibromyalgia and Environmental Illness by Burton Goldberg and The Editors Of Alternative Medicine Digest.

Alternative Medicine Guide – The Enzyme Cure by Lita Lee, Ph.D., Lisa Turner and With Burton Goldberg.

Alternative Medicine Guide To Heart Disease by Burton Goldberg and The Editors Of Alternative Medicine Digest.

Alternative Medicine Guide – Women's Health Series Books 1 and 2 by Burton Goldberg and The Editors Of Alternative Medicine Digest.

DHA: The Magnificent Marine Oil by Beth M. Ley Jacobs, Ph.D.

DMSO – Nature's Healer by Dr. Morton Walker.

Food Enzymes – The Missing Link To Radiant Health by Humbart Santillo, M.H., N.D.

Glucosamine, Nature's Arthritis Remedy by Ray Sahelian, M.D.

Omega-3 Oils – A Practical Guide by Donald Rudin, M.D. and Clara Felix.

Pain Free by Luke Bucci, Ph.D.

Reversing Fibromyalgia by Dr. Joe M. Elrod.

MSM: On Our Way Back To Health With Sulfur by Beth M. Ley.

Index

YOU NEED TO KNOW...
THE HEALTH MESSAGE